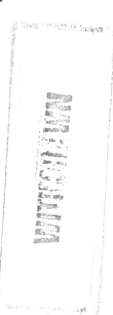

*Women helping women is the Wise Woman Way. The book you hold is a beautiful expression of this way. Read these women's stories and look into their faces. Let yourself be guided into that great metamorphosis we call menopause. This book will gladden your heart and enrich your mind. I recommend it highly.*

Susun S. Weed,
author of *New Menopausal Years the Wise Woman Way*

*Gabriele Kushi has a unique ability to see and inspire health and beauty. Her wisdom as a macrobiotic counselor, woven with the stories and images of many other women, makes this book an invaluable companion on the journey through the change of life.*

Nina Utne,
Chair, *Utne Magazine*

*This is the first book on menopause with a macrobiotic perspective. The stories illustrate many conditions women encounter during this change of life. The recipes will be of help for every woman's next stage of womanhood.*

Mayumi Nishimura,
Macrobiotic personal chef to Madonna

# Embracing Menopause

## *Naturally*

### Stories, Portraits and Recipes

## Gabriele Kushi

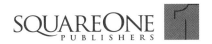
SQUAREONE
PUBLISHERS

Photography by © Gabriele Kushi. All rights reserved.
Except the photo of Aveline Kushi © Kushi Family Foundation; Brooke Medicine Eagle © Ann Wennhold; Marquita Wepman © Warren Wepman; Susun S. Weed © Susun S. Weed.

Photo of Gabriele Kushi © Jim Clifford
Cover photo © Gabriele Kushi
Book design: Randall Rogers and Jeannie Tudor
Typesetting: Theresa Wiscovitch
In-House Editor: Ariel Colletti
Interior Illustrations © Dagmar Goetzmann

**Square One Publishers**
115 Herricks Road
Garden City Park, NY 11040
(516) 535-2010 · (877) 900-BOOK
www.squareonepublishers.com

**Library of Congress Cataloging-in-Publication Data**
Kushi, Gabriele.
  Embracing menopause naturally : stories, portraits and recipes / Gabriele Kushi.
     p. cm.
  Includes bibliographical references and index.
  ISBN 0-7570-0296-X (pbk. : alk. paper)
1. Menopause—Psychological aspects. 2. Menopause—Diet therapy. 3. Macrobiotic diet—Recipes. 4. Menopause—Biography I. Title.

RG186.K87 2006
618.1'75—dc22
                                                    2006005846

Printed in the United States of America

10   9   8   7   6   5   4   3   2   1

# CONTENTS

*This book is lovingly dedicated*
*To my daughter Angelica, my mother Eleonore,*
*My mother-in-law Aveline, and her daughter Lily.*

Grandmother Bone
Give me strength.

The monthly blood
Soon will be gone.

Mother,
There must be
Something else?

*Gabriele Kushi*

# ACKNOWLEDGEMENTS

I would like to express my deepest appreciation to all the people who gave me support and encouragement for this book.

I am tremendously grateful to all the women who were courageous enough to share an intimate part of their lives with me, and from whom I learned so much. Without their encouragement and consent to publish their stories and photos in book form, this project would not have happened. These women are Aveline Kushi, Alice Red Elk, Brook Medicine Eagle, Carolyn Holbrook, Cecile Tovah Levin, Charlotte Anderson, Danielle Daniel, Darlene White Eagle, Diane Avoli, Dorothy Golden, Denise Wakefield Brave Hawk, Eve Blackwell, Hannah R. Weinberg, Isabelle Bird Horse, Jurate DiBenedetto, Laurie Savran, Lynn Marie Cross, Marquita Wepman, Monica Feifel, Rosangélica Aburto, Susun S. Weed, Sylvia Lemus Sharma, and Shizuko Yamamoto.

I also thank my artistic advisors Diane Katsiaficas, Joyce Lyon, and Jacquelyn Zita, who provided creative insights into the editing process of the photographs. I thank Patricia Thomas for her help in transcribing the audio-taped interviews of the women. My deep appreciation for her support in art, macrobiotics, and nutrition goes to Melinda Kizer, RD, and her family.

My heartfelt warmth is expressed to my first editor Carol Kozminski, from whom I also received the emotional support and affirmation of the importance of this book for menopausal women. Thanks to Molly Keating and Kelly Harth for their help with the editing process. My thanks and appreciation goes to my designer Randall Rogers for realizing my vision for the book. Special words of appreciation to my publisher, Rudy Shur, and everyone at Square One Publishers.

The remarkable illustrations of Dagmar Goetzmann are gratefully acknowledged. Special thanks to Anita Demands, Marie Olafsdaughter, Anne-Marie Fryer, Anna Merle, Gail Weber, and Richard Theobald for keeping me focused. My endless gratitude goes to Michio and Aveline Kushi, my in-laws and macrobiotic teachers. My deepest gratitude goes to Lawrence Haruo Kushi Sc. D., for his scientific guidance with this project, and our daughter Angelica Mariko, for her constant and loving support.

# FOREWORD

Women are the source and inspiration for great wisdom in the world that is passed from generation to generation. When they go through menopause and no longer give birth to children, they can direct more of their energy to nurturing their societies and communities. They can eventually become respected elders, with many years of experience and knowledge to give to others.

In this book, *Embracing Menopause Naturally*, Gabriele Kushi lets women speak about their experience with menopause. You can read how this change of life was for some women painful and emotional, and for others barely noticeable. But, for all women, it marked a time when their role in life had a major change. These seasoned women, rich in experiences, now give their wisdom to others while teaching younger women about this natural transition.

Gabriele was one of the first students to study macrobiotics at the Kushi Institute in Massachusetts, in 1978. She came from Germany and studied with many other international students. For many years now, her work has been to educate people about the macrobiotic natural way of life, through teaching cooking and counseling.

Women's health, photography, and cultural studies, have always been of great interest to Gabriele. When she first started to experience menopause symptoms, she became interested in how food and macrobiotics could influence menopause for her and other women. She researched the effects of food on women's health and hormones, and interviewed women from different cultural backgrounds about their experiences. Now, with this book *Embracing Menopause Naturally*, you can understand how these factors relate to each other. Gabriele also shares her favorite macrobiotic recipes for the midlife years.

This is the first book that looks at menopause and brings a macrobiotic perspective. I hope that it will be helpful for many women, and the men who are companions with them, in this important changing time in their lives.

Michio Kushi
Boston, Massachusetts
Author of *The Macrobiotic Path to Total Health*

# INTRODUCTION

## MY STORY

Surprised by my first hot flash, the need to connect to the earth mother's forgotten ancient symbols of menopausal women emerged, and ceremonies needed to be done.

Although it seemed too early, at forty-three, my menopausal passage had begun and lasted for five years. I found it curious that the end of my reproductive years and the beginning of my teenage daughter's should coincide. While collaborating with other women it became clear that what was happening in our family was happening in other families too.

As a macrobiotic consultant and cooking teacher who had lived a natural food lifestyle for many years, I understood the significance of food and its healing abilities in many physical imbalances. Naturally, I increased the amount of fermented soy foods and other plant hormonal regulators, like kale and daikon radish, when symptoms got too strong. I created new menus and taught Menopausal Cooking Classes. Some of my favorite recipes are included in this book.

When I was talking with my mother-in-law Aveline Kushi about her menopause, we wondered about other macrobiotic women's experiences with this passage. Aveline had devoted her life to sharing the macrobiotic way through cooking classes, and encouraging the growth and use of natural and organic whole foods all over the world. The inspiring autobiography *Aveline: The Life and Dream of the Woman Behind Macrobiotics Today* is a wonderful book about this remarkable woman and a continuation of her story.

While my menopause was in full throttle, I was completing my final work toward a BFA in Photography, Fine Arts, and Native American studies. My art always evolved around the feminine, and my intuition became stronger as my body changed. A desire to connect with menopausal women and to voice their experiences through photography and stories emerged. How did women who came from diverse cultural backgrounds experience this passage? Some of the women I searched for specifically, while others are friends or macrobiotic teachers and long-time acquaintances of mine. I designed a set of questions, the women had the freedom to answer or not, and this ethnographic study evolved over several years. As I explored my changes and came to know other women, the book *Embracing Menopause Naturally* took shape.

## ABOUT THE BOOK

*Embracing Menopause Naturally* concerns the time in a woman's life when some important experiences that have defined her life cease to be. The passage is a different experience for each woman, but it is a journey every woman must make. Awareness is the best preparation for what life has to offer. Becoming educated about menopause is important for women of all ages. Exploring options of how to handle symptoms is best started early, to find appropriate choices.

*Stories and Portraits of Menopausal Women* is the heart and soul of the book, and brings the diverse experiences and the beautiful faces of menopausal women to the reader. The women share where they were born and how many children and grandchildren they have. How and when they noticed their first menopausal symptoms, and what they did to alleviate them. Some turned to their traditional cultural rituals for affirmation of this phase of life, while others sought alternative or conventional medicine. Several already knew the benefits of macrobiotics, while others had changed their lifestyle as a result of menopause. The women share how the passage affected their quality of life and describe ways they have come to express their new selves.

Chapter One: *The Menopausal Passage* provides practical aspects of living with menopause. The hormonal changes during the phases of menopause and the role of phytoestrogens are discussed in relation to easing symptoms. Scientific research on Hormone Replacement Therapy and midlife issues relating to breast cancer, heart disease, and osteoporosis are discussed. Charts of herbs and natural foods rich in calcium and phytoestrogen, which have shown to address menopausal concerns, are designed for easy access.

Chapter Two: *Benefits of Macrobiotics for the Menopausal Passage* is a reminder to respond to the innate wisdom of embracing the menopausal passage by living in harmony with nature. A brief overview of macrobiotics is provided. Supported with research, macrobiotic guidelines enable women to make healthy choices for the midlife years and beyond. With these guidelines, a balanced meal plan can be easily integrated into any lifestyle.

Chapter Three: *Natural Food Recipes* provides menu suggestions for the midlife years. A wide variety of organic and natural ingredients provide phytoestrogens, minerals, vitamins, and proteins for a healthy lifestyle. Each recipe is balanced, and a varying formula is given to inspire your own creations with minimal effort.

I hope you enjoy this book as much as I enjoyed working with all the women. May it inspire and assist you in finding ways to truly make your passage a blessed one.

*Gabriele Kushi*
*www.kushiskitchen.com*

# ABOUT the STORIES and PORTRAITS of MENOPAUSAL WOMEN

My own menopausal passage sparked the interest in interviewing and photographing midlife women. I wanted to share the life experiences of other menopausal women and provide information for this important time in a woman's life. My experience in teaching macrobiotics internationally, in large group situations as well as one-on-one, has given me the cornerstone for my collaborative work with the women.

When I first started asking my women friends what they thought menopause was, some of them did not have clear ideas, whereas others were dealing with the change very effectively. My German friend Monica Feifel said she had started her menopausal journey and takes estrogen to alleviate her hot flashes, but would like to try more natural ways. Laurie Savran had increased her exercise and tried to eat better. Lynn Marie Cross, my long-time macrobiotic friend, just started using wild yam cream to control her hot flashes. For me, hot flashes were like sweat lodges where the body purifies itself of excess energy it no longer needs.

The women I talked to who had not yet entered the journey, and had not educated themselves about menopause, had mostly negative associations with it. Some identified it with old age, which dries one up from the inside out, like an old prune. They thought it meant being over the hill, not being attractive anymore. Michelle said, "I am happy with my monthly cycles and I feel young and attractive." Then she made a cross with her hands over her face as if she wanted to ward off menopause. I thought sadly, if only that would help to fight it off.

For this project I chose women from a diversity of cultures to explore universal approaches to menopause. Most of the women I was introduced to specifically in the context of this project, while others I had known for a long time. Some of the stories are based on interviews, while others are stories written in their own words. The whole process of contacting, interviewing, editing the

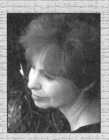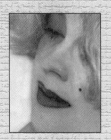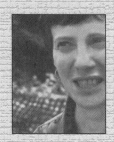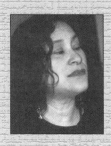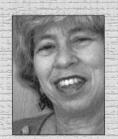

stories, and photographing the women lasted for several years. A camera and a tape recorder were my constant companions.

With the portraits of the women, I add a visual image to each woman's voice, the perceptible synthesis of the woman's experience of her menopausal passage. The predominant focus in my art is to create sacred spaces and rituals for the feminine. My art has developed over the years in this way and I receive strength and fulfillment from it. Sometimes when I made the photos of the women at the same time I did the interview, an intense dynamic developed, which was very invigorating. When I just photographed the woman, and she gave me the story at a separate time, a more quiet interaction happened.

I asked the women to consider the following nine questions while voicing their menopausal story. Some of the woman tried to answer all the questions, while others concentrated on only one or two aspects.

What are the general experiences of your menopausal passage? What do you want people to learn from your experience? Did you use conventional or holistic approaches for symptom relief? What were the effects of the menopausal passage on relationships or quality of work? How are

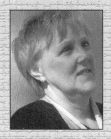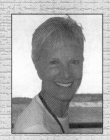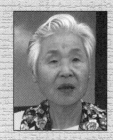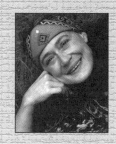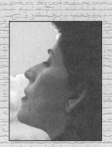

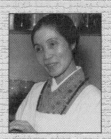 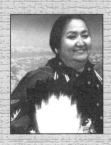 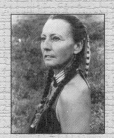 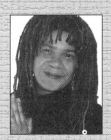 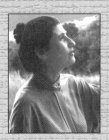

menopausal women viewed in your community? How do the women view themselves? How do children and grandchildren affect the quality of midlife? Is there a new way of expressing one's self as a midlife woman? How are creative impulses realized?

The variety of experiences in the stories of the women's menopausal passages contains valid information and illustrates what could be expected while going through menopause. The women create a supportive community for the reader—whether she is a woman who is encountering menopause, a woman interested in what menopause entails, or a man searching for insight about a woman he cares for. Menopause is not to be dreaded, but accepted as a continuation of a woman's evolution. Menopause offers opportunities for a woman to grow spiritually, live healthfully and become aware of her needs, physically and emotionally.

As you read through the book, you will find different stories at the beginning of each chapter. Judgment is placed neither on the experiences of the women, nor on how they have dealt with their menopause. Aveline's story is placed at the beginning to honor her place in my life.

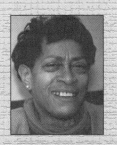 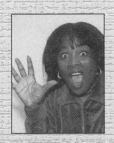 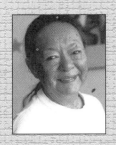 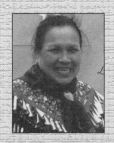 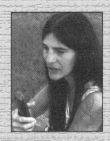

# STORIES and PORTRAITS

*Aveline Kushi*

*Alice Red Elk*

*Brooke Medicine Eagle*

*Carolyn Holbrook*

*Cecile Tovah Levin*

# AVELINE KUSHI

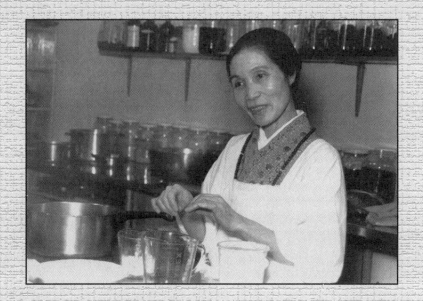

$\mathcal{I}$ was born in Japan but lived most of my adult life in the U.S.A. I am the mother of five children and the grandmother of fourteen.

Menopause might be difficult for some women, but I did not notice it that way. I heard that many women have menopause problems like hot flashes, or problems with their husbands. But I think it will all become much more peaceful after menopause. You will see.

After my monthly cycle ceased, I experienced a deep peaceful feeling, which I never had before in my life. It was so beautiful. It made me enjoy life more. I was fifty-three years old when my periods became irregular. It took about five years for my menstruation to stop completely.

In 1950 at age twenty-six, I began studying macrobiotics and started eating brown rice, miso soup and vegetables. This food was dramatically different from my previous diet of white rice, sugar treats and raw foods. To my surprise my menstruation stopped. With no boyfriend at that time, I did not worry that I was pregnant. I was only astonished at how my body was changing. After nine months, my menstruation came back. It lasted three days and then stopped. Before macrobiotics, I usually had heavy menstruation, but because of my good diet, my periods became clean, easy, and short. This pause of the menstrual cycle occurs sometimes when women start a wholesome way of eating. However, it is nothing to worry about. The wholesome food cleans and heals the vital organs of the body first, before revitalizing the sexual organs, so periods can become healthy and regular.

When I grew up in Japan, I never heard elderly people talk about menopause. But then I never knew my grandmother, only my grandfather, and I never talked about that with him. I remember in college a classmate's mother could not stop bleeding for over 10 days. In retrospect, I realized that her mother probably was going through menopause.

Ten years ago, I was in Munich at a macrobiotic conference. At a women's discussion group, I was asked how to handle menopausal symptoms. I was about to answer, when a lady in the back raised her hand and spoke. "If you have any problem with menopause," she said, "don't eat any animal foods, eggs, milk, or cheese. Eliminate all sweets, chocolate, and fruits. If you still have problems, instead of eating three meals per day eat only two. If you still have trouble, eat only once per day and if you still have trouble, don't eat at all. These were my grandmother's suggestions. I followed them and I did not have any problems."

I was really happy to listen to her story, because I wanted to give the same suggestions. The menopausal passage is a big part of a woman's life cycle. It can feel like a tremendous tornado passing through. But don't worry and try not to escape. Just observe it. Maybe hide in a cave till the tornado passes and adjust any problem day to day with food.

# ALICE HEHÄKA' LÙTA (RED ELK)

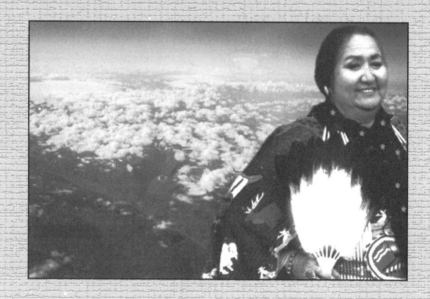

$\mathcal{I}$ am from the Standing Rock Lakota Reservation in Fort Yates, North Dakota. I am a mother of five, with four daughters, one son, and thirteen grandchildren, including two sets of female twins.

I want to say a few things about the change that went through my whole being. Anatomy and physiology tell us that menopause affects all women between ages forty-five and fifty. During this time, our bodies stop producing hormones and our ovaries stop producing eggs, so we can no longer become pregnant. During this time our thinking also changes.

Without the creator in my life, I know I would never have dealt with it properly. For native women, this is where our traditions come into play. During hot flashes, there are certain ceremonies we do. We burn sage and Azi'liciup—smudge ourselves to help alleviate certain pressures.

The process of menopause became a spiritual journey. My whole physical, mental, and spiritual self changed. The change that came to help my thinking was a spiritual experience that took me to a different place. It is a place where no one, or no thing, can bother or touch me. To be able to achieve this spiritual feeling, I needed to learn to love and honor the Great Spirit and be able to give back in terms of love. Spiritually I am able to give my love with more depth, not only to Native women but also to my fellow men.

Through the Grandmother's Society, I work with Native women in the prison system. This helps me to express and identify myself as a whole spiritual being in my postmenopausal state. Being more loving, compassionate, and humble brings about a great creativity, which I express by doing fine art work, or dancing at a traditional Native American Pow-Wow. Creativity can take many forms, and it all comes from the creator. Mi Takuye Oya'sin. To all my relations.

# BROOKE MEDICINE EAGLE

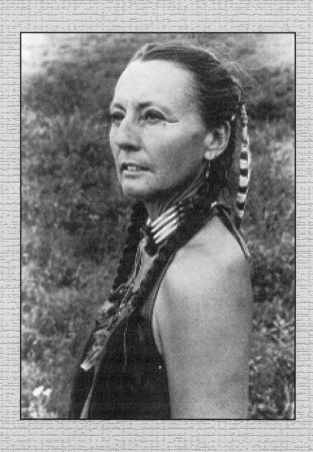

*I* was raised on the Crow Reservation in Montana where my father was born. My parents were of mixed blood ancestry, which included several native tribes and European lineages. This background gave me an interest in the healing ways common to all people on Earth. I have no children of my own, but my Native tradition says if you have no children, then all children are yours.

The understanding about the wisdom years of the menopausal (Moon-Pause) woman is generic to most cultures. The current American culture had largely forgotten this vital knowledge, until some of us began to bring the ancient wisdom forward again.

I experienced menarche at fourteen in total ignorance and embarrassment. Since then I have rediscovered the ancient ways of my mother's Lakota heritage. I learned about one of the seven sacred rites, called Her Alone They Sing Over—when a girl who reached menarche was highly honored in the center of a celebration of continuing life. The touch of the new maiden was said to convey wonderful life energy to all around her. Many women, including myself, had not received this knowledge at menarche, and were deeply healed by being recipients of the honoring ceremony, notwithstanding its being performed forty years late.

My periods were always regular, light and without challenge. At fifty-five, I became peri-menopausal with a similar lack of complication. One month, I spotted; the next, I bled profusely; the month after, there was no period. After several months, I understood that that part of my life was complete. My sadness came from learning about the power and mystery of women's blood so late in life. I had little time to come into harmony with my moon cycles and consciously step beyond the veil into the wisdom that awaited women during menopause.

For most of my life, I experienced low kidney energy and constant coolness in my body. When I warmed up during menopause, I actually welcomed it. My female naturopath worked with me to balance my body during this time of change. Eating well and taking a few homeopathic supplements made all the difference for me, although memory challenges continue to plague me.

It is an honor to be in the Grandmother Wisdom Lodge, and yet, I am not feeling as wise as I think some traditional women might have felt. Tribal women had a lifetime of preparation. They went each month into their moon lodges for four days of rest, quiet, and meditation. There, they vision-quested more than anyone else in the world. One can see how they became wise. Imagine four hundred and fifty quests of four days, by the time of Moon Pause! This kind of devotion and supported journeying to bring forth information for the people, truly created wisdom.

To share the teachings of the Wisdom Lodge with other women in this critical and powerful transition on Earth is very important to me. We wisdom women learn to gather our power to teach the ways of nurturing good relationships to those around us. Love and Power, which will truly transform the Earth, will spread and become the primary energy. All life will be served!

# CAROLYN HOLBROOK

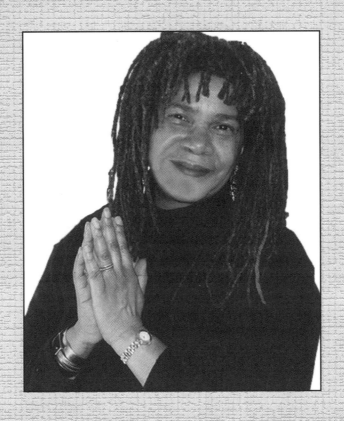

*I* have five children and six grandchildren.

All the symptoms of menopause found in textbooks—hot flashes, vaginal dryness, night sweats, insomnia, mood swings, depression, and weight gain—I have experienced. Because of my belief in natural medicines, I was reluctant to take Hormone Replacement Therapy. The herbal remedies Dong Quai and Black Cohosh were helpful for some symptoms, but not my insomnia, which became unbearable. Finally, I was given the hormone Premarin at a women's medical clinic. This raised my blood pressure to an unhealthy level and caused my legs to cramp.

A well-known woman doctor who specializes in menopause explained that some women simply do not fare well on Premarin and suggested I use the Estroderm patch. My ancestral African mothers used herbal remedies for all kinds of ailments and I honor their wisdom. But my doctor discouraged combining herbal medicines with traditional Western remedies.

After more disappointing visits and months of searching, I finally found a doctor who listened carefully to my concerns. He respected that a woman who had lived long enough to experience menopause knew her own body. He prescribed a gentler form of the Estrogen patch and referred me to an Alternative Health Clinic. On my next visit he checked my estrogen level and determined that the combination of herbs, acupuncture, and the Estrogen patch was working. Because of my sensitivity to medicines, it was the right thing to combine traditional and non-traditional treatments. I felt better than I had felt in years.

As a young woman, I would have been too intimidated to search for a doctor with whom I felt comfortable. Now, I have no qualms about speaking up for myself. I know who I am and am finally comfortable with myself.

There is a depth to my creativity that wasn't there before. My thoughts flow like the River Nile. I find great joy in sharing whatever wisdom I have attained with my three daughters and other young women. I continue to discover new things about myself, as I grow older. Unlike my earlier years, there is less anxiety accompanying these discoveries. Instead, there is a feeling of well-being.

# CECILE TOVAH LEVIN

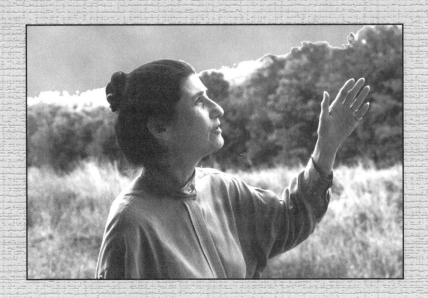

*I* was born in the United States, where I raised my two children on my own.

My menopause started a few months shy of forty-nine years. I experienced hot flashes during the night. Fortunately, I had been macrobiotic for twenty-six years and that helped me go through menopause quite comfortably. I could keep my body energy balanced by increasing green and white vegetables, which kept my hot flash temperature down. Hot flashes arise from hormone re-balancing and also from excessive liver heat, which can be triggered by stress. Increasing intake of sea vegetables like hiziki and arame helped to re-balance the hormonal secretions. I stopped eating animal foods.

Macrobiotics is the original way of life that supports ecological, biological, and physiological life systems on earth. The grasses, trees, animals, and birds live according to universal laws, natural laws. Human beings have strayed from these natural laws and therefore have physical and mental illness. This balanced macrobiotic way of life is brought into modern memory through teaching and cooking. Because food plays such an essential role in health and happiness, cooking really is the highest art and the highest responsibility for human beings to take on. We have the power in our hands and in our kitchens to change our destiny.

I have always lived close to nature and the universal laws. My home has been a macrobiotic healing and educational center. I have helped many people—male and female, old and young—pass through crises of physical illness and psychological difficulty. That is very creative, because one must be in touch with the life force, physically, emotionally, and spiritually, to guide other people. When one is teaching and helping to heal others, one is also teaching and healing one's self. I have used this opportunity to develop my teaching and writing skills, and returned to creating artwork, which I had given up before childbirth.

After the period of hot flashes, I felt sad to be losing the possibility of increasing my family, which had been a dream of mine. This sadness ceased when I recognized menopause as a passage into a higher realm of self, where energies are reabsorbed into the body toward cultivation of wisdom.

Menopause gives women the opportunity to refine that energy into a spiritual quality. The ultimate goal is the growth of women to become mentors of the younger generation, to guide them toward health, happiness, peace, and spiritual development. I think menopause is the opening door, a gateway to a higher level of life. It happens at the appropriate time in a woman's life to continue to the next stage of human development. It should not be regarded as a sickness, but as a sacred passage.

# CHAPTER ONE
# THE MENOPAUSAL PASSAGE

## THE VIEW ON MENOPAUSE

For generations the menopausal passage has not been addressed correctly. Myth, fear, and misconceptions painted a negative picture of menopause. As a result, many women are afraid of it. Sigmund Freud, for instance, described menopausal women as "quarrelsome, peevish, and argumentative, petty and miserly..." Psychiatrist Dr. David Reuben declared that after menopause, a woman becomes "not really a man but no longer a functional woman" in his best-selling book, *Everything You Always Wanted to Know About Sex, But Were Afraid to Ask.*[2] In a time when plastic surgery supports a youth and sex-obsessed society, middle age does not even seem to exist.

When women are actually asked about their experiences with menopause, the vast majority does not have experiences that live up to these negative characterizations. Drs. Sonja and John McKinlay of the New England Research Institute interviewed 2,300 women who were approaching or passing through menopause to find out how it affected their physical and psychological health.[3] The results showed that only 3 percent of the 2,300 women expressed regret during or after menopause about the physical changes associated with menopause. Few lamented the end of menstruation and many, according to the study, felt relieved about not having to worry about contraception, menstruation and pregnancy. Some of the women I interviewed for this book expressed these same feelings. Dr. Christiane Northrup, a well-known gynecologist and diligent advocate for women's health, states in her book *Women's Wisdom, Women's Bodies,* that 80 percent of women do not experience menopause as a problem, although society does, because of our ageist and sexist culture.

Can a woman's status in her society influence the way she experiences her change of life, her menopause? Ann Rite's study revealed that there is a difference in how traditional and non-traditional Navajo women experience their menopause. The traditional women had fewer symptoms of menopause. The reason seems to be that traditional Navajo people know that the changes in nature are connected with the changing cycles of women. The !Kung women, from the traditional tribe living in Africa, do not even have a word for hot flash, suggesting that these symptoms are not experienced, or are experienced as a natural and accepted part of change.[4]

In traditional Native American cultures there has always been celebration when a woman entered menarche and menopause. Special tasks and responsibilities came to her when she reached menopause. "When a woman reached menopause she frequently received the power, from medicine men or from vision, to engage in various rituals," writes Marla N. Powers in her book *Oglala Women*. In ancient times, postmenopausal women became wise women of their culture, the seeds of wisdom.

Women are changing western-society views about menopausal women and the meaning of midlife. Acceptable and non-judgmental language about women's issues declare menopause as a meaningful passage into old age. Women are beginning to discover what menopause really means, and reconsider covering it up through face-lifts. They are aware of the risks of Hormone Replacement Therapy, and want to experience a natural menopause. Through balanced diets with regular exercise women stop worrying that their bodies are going to disintegrate, their hearts are going to dissolve, and their bones are going to break. Women are networking with other women and sharing experiences to avoid feeling isolated and find beauty and value in life. Women experience menopause with awareness. They are taking the initiation into wisdom and honor themselves. They tell the truth about what they are feeling, and stand up for what they believe. To bring forth such motion is imperative in women's personal lives, as well as in the political sector. Not only will society's view of women change; women will bring a sense of balance and healing to the planet.

# WHAT IS MENOPAUSE?

*Menopause* is the time when a woman passes from her childbearing years. It is a natural passage, just like *menarche*—the onset of menstruation—and pregnancy. Menopause literally means stop of menstruation, and it marks the time when menstruation and the fertility cycles have ceased for one year. One talks about a passage, because to arrive at the state of menopause, the body often needs time to prepare and adjust.

## Menopausal Symptoms

Hot flashes, emotional upheaval, crankiness, restlessness, irritability, depression, insomnia, migraines, irregular periods, dry vagina, loss of libido, weight gain, and digestive problems can all be signs that the body is preparing for menopause.

The process of hormonal adjustment during the menopausal passage can last from two to fifteen years. The time and symptoms of the passage depend on the overall physical, mental, spiritual, and emotional condition of a woman. When the hormonal adjustment process is finally over, menopausal symptoms generally cease. In the menopausal stories, the most common symptoms expressed were irregular periods, digestive problems, and hot flashes.

## Ways to Ease
## Menopausal Symptoms Naturally

Maintain a constant blood sugar level
Do regular and moderate exercises like Yoga
Perform daily deep breathing and relaxation techniques
Eat moderate and balanced natural food meals
Eliminate all hot flash triggers

## HOT FLASH VISUALIZATION

Visualize being outside in the depth of winter when the land is covered with snow and the cold, freezing wind takes your breath away. You come inside the warm and cozy house and drink a hot cup of tea or eat a hot stew. A feeling of warmth comes over you, and suddenly you sweat and have to quickly take off your sweater. Now imagine that even without drinking that hot cup, you experience three or four such sweats within one hour. They may even wake you in the middle of the night. These are the sensations of *hot flashes*—sudden rushes of hot energy that spread upward to the neck and head, lasting anywhere from thirty seconds to five minutes.

Hot flashes can feel like *sweat lodges*—Native American rituals where the body purifies itself of excess energy. Worldwide, 570 million women are going through menopause, and seventy-five percent of them experience hot flashes.

## HOT FLASH TRIGGERS

**The following foods with predominant Yin (expanding) energy can trigger hot flashes:**

Citrus fruits, tomatoes, strawberries, chocolate, spicy foods such as chilies, hot liquids with or without caffeine, and alcohol, especially wine.

Hot and humid weather, a warm bed, clothing made of synthetic fibers (which inhibit breathability), stress, anxiety, strenuous exercises, meals eaten too quickly, and overeating or eating large meals.

**Other conditions that can trigger hot flashes.**

**The following foods with predominant Yang (contracting) energy can trigger hot flashes:**

All kinds of meat, eggs, hard cheeses, chips, and popcorn.

# THE TRANSFORMATIONAL PROCESS

The medical community has divided the *climacteric*—menopause, popularly known as change of life—into three stages: peri-menopause, menopause, and post-menopause. The first stage, *peri-menopause*, marks the beginning of the transition and can last about four years before and two years after the final menstrual cycle. Those are the years women notice the most physical changes, such as irregular periods and hot flashes.

*Menopause*, the second stage, occurs when one has not had a period for one year. Therefore, it can only be identified in retrospect.

The third stage, the *post-menopausal years*, is the rest of a women's life after her final period. Margaret Mead describes the post-menopausal years as a time of a renewed sense of self and increased vitality and zest.

The three stages of menopause are not very clear-cut, especially when passing through them, and can be determined only in retrospect. Also, the symptoms a woman experiences can overlap across these three stages. The changes a woman goes through during these years can be very profound on all levels of her being. The effect can be felt not only by herself, but also by her family and eventually her community.

The average age of menopause is fifty-one, but the changes can be felt as early as age thirty-eight.[5] Occurrence before the age of thirty-five is generally considered premature. Menopause is considered late when it begins after age fifty-five. If your menopause has not started soon after this age, there is no cause for alarm. You should, however, check with your health care provider, because there may be an increased risk of uterine and breast cancer due to prolonged exposure to your body's own estrogen. Menopause can be brought on through surgical removal of the ovaries, chemotherapy, radiation, tubal ligation, mumps, an autoimmune reaction, extreme stress, and weight loss.

A natural menopausal passage, which can last from two to fifteen years, is a transformational process, a letting go of the old self with a rebirth of a new self. One can divide the passage of menopause into three spiritual stages: isolation, death, and rebirth. If a woman sees menopause as an initiation, then she can draw inward for a period of time and isolate herself. Then, the signs of hot flashes, headaches, and emotional outbursts become allies of wholeness instead of a problem. The death, seen as the ripping away of the old, can become a period of mourning and desperation. The rebirth is seen as a total metamorphosis to a new self. If a woman chooses to experience menopause in this natural way, said Tamara Slayton, she is empowered to fulfill her life's mission after completion of these three spiritual stages.

## THE HORMONAL CYCLE

The *endocrine system* regulates most of the hormonal activity in a female body. *Estrogen* and *progesterone* are the main hormones involved in a woman's fertility cycle. Estrone, estradiol, and estriol are all natural forms of estrogen, produced primarily by the ovaries, adrenal glands, fat cells, placenta and fetus. Each month, *Follicle Stimulating Hormones (FSH)* and *Luteinizing Hormones (LH)* are produced to assist the ovaries in the fertilization process of an egg. When a woman is in her mid-thirties, the ovaries start to produce less estradiol. When menstruation finally stops, the levels of estrogen produced in the ovaries are drastically reduced, although the ovaries never completely stop producing estrogen.

The fat cells in a woman's body also produce estrogen through the conversion of androstenedione. The adrenal glands secrete androstenedione into the bloodstream, and it is converted into estrogen in the fat cells, liver, and kidney.[6] This process assures some women with normal weight an easier transition through menopause. Thus going on a weight (fat)-loss diet is not advisable for a menopausal woman, because she might increase her menopausal symptoms, although extreme excessive weight and high refined carbohydrate and saturated fat intake is unhealthy.

Progesterone is produced primarily by the adrenal glands and by the ovarian corpus luteum during a woman's ovulatory years. When pregnant, progesterone is also produced by the placenta. As ovulation slows and ceases during the menopausal years, progesterone levels fall. Most sixty-year-old women have little or no progesterone. Progesterone and estrogen are also critical hormones in bone formation.[7]

When the ovulatory cycle ceases, Follicle Stimulating Hormones often start to accumulate in the system. The liver has to do extra work to digest this overload of hormones, which sometimes slows the general digestive process. A healthy body with strong energy in the liver, kidney, and spleen is of utmost importance at this time.

## RISKS OF HORMONE REPLACEMENT THERAPY

Blood tests or saliva hormone level testing can be done to determine estrogen and progesterone levels. However, if estrogen and progesterone levels are low, doctors may recommend *Hormone Replacement Therapy (HRT)*, sometimes without discussing the risks or offering other options.

Carolyn Holbrook mentioned in her story that she was given HRT but did not feel well using it. She had to change her physician several times to find someone sensitive to her needs, to combine holistic and conventional medicine.

Estrogen Replacement Therapy came to the market in the 1960s. This was done without much testing. The major estrogen that is available and usually prescribed is made from the urine of a pregnant mare. These mares are kept artificially pregnant to produce the estrogen needed to manufacture the drug Premarin (pregnant-mare-urine). Synthetically formulated estrogen is also available. In the 1990s, estrogen became the second most prescribed drug in America.

Hormone Replacement Therapy not only increases a woman's risk of breast cancer, but produces a more aggressive form of cancer and delays detection of tumors. According to a study published in 2003 in the *Journal of the American Medical Association*, these factors make it less likely that the cancer will be cured.

These findings suggest that HRT is beneficial only for short-term use, and under restricted circumstances. Dr. Susan Hendrix of Wayne State University, Detroit, one of the authors of the study, hopes that these findings will convince women of the disadvantages of HRT. Dr. Peter H. Gann and Dr. Monica Morrow of Northwestern University commented, "The message for physicians caring for menopausal patients is clear. The results of the Dr. Susan Hendrix study provide further compelling evidence against the use of combination estrogen plus progestin hormone therapy."

Hormone Replacement Therapy has been widely used in menopausal women because of the belief that the treatment not only eases hot flashes and other acute symptoms of menopause, but also increases bone density, protects against heart disease and stroke, and delays the onset of dementia.

In the years 2002 and 2003, however, those beliefs were entirely overturned, largely as a result of the Women's Health Initiative, a massive study of more than 16,000 women. That study was ended prematurely in 2002 when it became clear that HRT increased the risk of breast cancer while providing no benefit against heart disease and stroke. In May 2003, further analysis from that study found that HRT also does not protect against dementia.

**Risks of Hormone Replacement Therapy**

**1.** Women who use HRT are more likely to develop cardiovascular diseases, including heart disease. This is definitely true for *combination therapy*, combining estrogen with progestin; whether this is true for estrogens alone is currently being studied, but estrogens alone are known to increase the chances of developing breast and uterine cancer.

**2.** Women who use HRT are more likely to have dementia and cognitive decline. This has been demonstrated for combination therapy. Whether this is true for estrogens alone is currently being studied.

**3.** HRT produces a more aggressive form of cancer and delays the detection of breast cancer cells.

A team headed by Dr. Hendrix and Dr. Rowan T. Chlebowski of Harbor-UCLA in Los Angeles examined the data from the Women's Health Initiative. The researchers found that women taking the hormones had 24 percent higher risk of breast cancer compared with women taking a placebo; there were about eight extra cases for every 10,000 women taking HRT. At diagnosis, tumors were larger in the women taking hormones. Moreover, the tumors had begun to spread to 25.4 percent of hormone users, compared with only 16 percent of those receiving placebos.

Genes, family history, blood pressure, diet, environment, and many unknown variables must be considered when considering HRT. The decision process must be separated from the fear, and it can be difficult to choose which direction to pursue. If threatening images of wrinkled women, robbed of sexual drive, depressed, or crippled with osteoporosis are the only guide a women has, her fear factors will unfortunately rise. The women I interviewed for this book urge you to counter such fears through exercise and sound nutrition.

## EMBRACING MENOPAUSE NATURALLY

A balanced diet and exercise have been proven to be positive choices not only for women dealing with menopause, but also for those dealing with midlife issues like heart disease, osteoporosis, and cancer. Testimonies from women and recommendations from medical doctors sympathetic to holistic health care confirm the findings of researchers: with a holistic and natural food lifestyle, the menopausal passage can be eased.

Dr. Christiane Northrup recommends combining a grain-based diet rich in foods that contain plant-estrogens with exercise for menopause as well as for a strong heart, healthy bones, and decreased risk of cancer.[8] The stories of many women confirm the importance of natural food and a balanced lifestyle in dealing with menopause.

Studies have shown that just one serving of soy each day (a half cup of tofu) reduces hot flashes by 10 to 20 percent. It is also a well-known fact that the frequency of symptoms of menopause are lower in Asia than in America. The reasons for this seem to be the low-fat and high-fiber Asian diet, and the consumption of traditional soy products such as miso and tofu from an early age, both of which are less common for American women.[9]

One of the reasons a plant-based natural food diet is believed to be beneficial for the menopausal woman is that the phytoestrogens from eating plant-based foods can stimulate estrogen-like effects in the body. This is possible because the chemical structures of these phytoestrogens (such as the isoflavones, daidzein, or genistein) are similar to the structures of the estrogens made by the body (estradiol). Although these phytoestrogens are considerably weaker than one's own estrogens, they can compete for the same estrogen receptors and may ease menopausal symptoms, including hot flashes.

Therapies such as homeopathy, aromatherapy, herbal medicine, acupuncture, acupressure, therapeutic touch, shiatsu, and self-massage are excellent methods to support a balanced natural food lifestyle and to embrace menopause naturally.

# NATURAL FOODS RICH IN PHYTOESTROGENS FOR THE MENOPAUSAL PASSAGE

*Phytoestrogens*—plant-estrogens—are a class of compounds found in plants that, in humans, have a similar effect to estrogen. Phytoestrogens include such compounds as isoflavones, lignans, and coumestans. Soybeans and red clover are the principle sources of isoflavones; mung beans, alfalfa, and soy sprouts are the main sources of coumestans; and flaxseed is a particularly rich source of lignans. The content of phytoestrogens in food varies depending on how and where the food is grown.

Studies have shown that eating soy and other food rich in phytoestrogen is a healthy choice. However, recently developed soy foods manufactured from soy protein isolates, such as soy beverages or imitation meats and cheeses, are not always the best choices. Isolated soy protein, once considered a waste product with an offensive odor, has been transformed with flavorings, preservatives, sweeteners, emulsifiers, and synthetic chemicals into a questionable product for human consumption.[10]

**Phytoestrogen-Rich Natural Foods**

Soybeans, flaxseed, linseed, rye, most whole grains, mung beans, alfalfa sprouts, and red clover. Foods containing smaller amounts of phytoestrogens include collards, kale, cabbage, broccoli, and berries.

Consider including traditional soy foods in your meal plan. Non-genetically modified whole soybeans are best eaten fermented as miso, soy sauce, tamari, tempeh, or natto. The fresh green soybean—edamame—can be eaten as an appetizer, steamed and seasoned with sea salt. Tofu, a non-fermented soybean product, should mainly be consumed seasoned with fermented tamari soy sauce or miso.

| SUBSTANCE | CLAIMED EFFECTS |
| --- | --- |
| Tofu | Relieves hot flashes; Provides phytoestrogen |
| Soy Sauce, Tamari | Aid digestion |
| Miso, Natto, Tempeh | Provide enzymes and phytoestrogens |
| Sea Vegetables | Build bones; Provide vitamins and minerals |
| Leafy Green Vegetables | Relieve hot flashes; Build bones; Provide vitamins and minerals |
| Seeds | Provide phytoestrogen; Moisturize tissue |
| Whole Grains | Provide phytoestrogen; Build bones |
| Gomasio, Ume-Sho-Bancha | Relieve cramps |
| Charred Umeboshi Plum | Minimizes excess menstrual bleeding |

## HERBS FOR THE MENOPAUSAL PASSAGE

Herbs rich in plant sterols—*phytosterols*—also have estrogen-like effects, and are another choice to reduce menopausal symptoms, according to Susun Weed, the author of *New Menopausal Years the Wise Woman Way*. Some of these herbs are raspberry leaf, sage leaf, dandelion root, ginseng root, motherwort flowering top, chaste tree berry, nettle leaf, and black cohosh root. These herbs, Weed recommends, are best taken as infusions or tinctures, and not in capsules.

A scientific study was done in 1988 in Germany on the effects of the plant sterol-rich herb black cohosh. The test results showed that black cohosh is as effective as Estrogen Replacement Therapy in reducing the menopausal symptoms of hot flashes, headaches, joint pain, water retention, and fatigue. This was documented both objectively in tests of hormone levels, and subjectively in the reports by the women tested. Studies are underway in the US to replicate these findings.

To ease hot flashes one can also use a mixture of the Chinese herbs, which includes dong quai and ginseng. Dong quai is taken by Chinese women most often to improve female conditions. Dong quai contains plant sterols that can have strong estrogen-like effects, but only if digested well and eaten with fermented foods such as yogurt or miso.

Choosing to experience menopause naturally with plant-based meals rich in phytoestrogens and phytosterol-rich herbs seems to be an option for women who don't want to be exposed to the risk of breast cancer due to Hormone Replacement Therapy. Some plants and herbs have estrogenic qualities, but studies have not yet been conclusive as to how much and how often these foods need to be eaten to deter or prevent breast cancer. As a whole, dietary phytoestrogens and phytosterol-rich herbs are associated with a lower risk of heart disease, cancer, and osteoporosis, and assist in easing some menopausal symptoms.

**Herbs for the Menopausal Passage**

Raspberry leaf, sage leaf, dandelion root, ginseng root, motherwort flowering top, chaste tree berry, nettle leaf, and black cohosh root.

# MIDLIFE ISSUES ASSOCIATED with MENOPAUSE

## BREAST CANCER

The body produces its own estrogens, which are needed for normal reproduction. The risk of breast cancer increases with increased exposure to the body's own estrogens (estradiol). This exposure may be caused by having few or no pregnancies, early menstruation or late menopause, a first pregnancy at a later age, or not breast feeding. Being exposed to external estrogens, including through Estrogen or Hormone Replacement Therapy, environmental estrogens, and estrogen consumed in foods, can also increase the risk of breast cancer.

A high intake of foods like miso and whole grains seems to suppress the body's production of the estrogen that feeds hormone-dependent cancers.[11] Theoretically, the consumption of high-quality vegetables that contain phytoestrogens can block and thus may reduce the cancer-causing estrogen's ability to bind with the cell.

Researchers have found that genistein, which is found in soy, is capable of inhibiting the growth of a wide range of cancer cells.[12] Data presented in a review of studies entitled *Soy Intake and Cancer Risk* indicates that protection may extend to breast, prostate, and colon cancer. Studies, however, caution women who already have estrogen-dependent breast cancer or those with a past history of it against starting to consume large amounts of phytoestrogens from soy.

A study of women published in the *International Journal of Cancer* (2005) revealed that eating beans at least twice per week could help reduce the risk of chronic conditions, including heart disease and certain types of cancer.[13] The high protein and fiber content, folates, minerals, and other phytochemicals in beans may explain their cancer-fighting powers. Good choices include kidney beans, black beans, chickpeas, navy beans, adzuki beans, lentils, soybeans, and peas. This study, which included 90,000 women aged twenty-six to forty-six, revealed that those who consumed two or more servings of beans per week had a reduced risk of breast cancer compared to those who consumed beans less than once a month.

To increase beans in your diet, substitute them for foods that are high in saturated fat, such as red meat or other animal-based proteins. Start by reducing the amount of meat required for any dish and adding beans to the recipe. Choose bean dips as healthy alternatives to sour cream or cream cheese dips and spreads.

## HEART DISEASE

Heart disease is the number one cause of death among postmenopausal women in the US. This probably has little correlation to menopause and is more a result of the aging process. However, there are a number of things that women can do to decrease the likelihood of developing heart disease. The most important ones are regular physical activity, a heart-healthy diet, and not smoking.

To choose a diet that promotes heart health, one should emphasize plant-based foods. Whole grains, fresh vegetables, fruits, beans, and legumes should be the mainstays of the diet. Animal foods, especially those high in saturated fats and cholesterol, should be minimized or avoided. One should also avoid foods with trans fatty acids.

Almost all trans fatty acids are created in commercial food processing through *hydrogenation*. Hydrogenation transforms vegetable oils into fats that are more stable and thus prolong the shelf life of foods. However, trans fatty acids are known to dramatically increase the risk of heart disease. It is easy to avoid trans fatty acids by reading food labels. Any product that contains hydrogenated or partially hydrogenated oils or fats will also contain trans fatty acids.

Omega-3 fatty acids have been shown to have a positive effect on preventing cardiovascular disease and maintaining cardiovascular health. These fats are not only important for heart health, but for every cell in the body. People deficient in omega-3 fatty acids may experience fatigue, dry skin, cracked nails, thin and breakable hair, constipation, immune system malfunction, aching joints, depression, arthritis, and hormonal imbalances. Many of these symptoms are often associated with menopause.

These fatty acids are found in flaxseed and fatty fish such as salmon, albacore, herring, and mackerel. Cod liver oil, egg yolk, and algae are other possible sources. Flaxseed oil, with its composition of 57-percent omega-3 fatty acids, served cold with a dressing over salads, is a palatable choice. Another choice is $1/4$ cup of ground flaxseed three to seven days a week. Grind your daily serving in a coffee grinder. Stir the flax meal into soups, beverages, cereals, or salads. The flax meal must be prepared fresh daily, due to its high rate of oxidation.

**Flaxseed Mixture**

1 teaspoon pumpkin seeds and 1 teaspoon flax seeds
Preparation: Grind seeds in a little grinder and serve immediately.
Sprinkle over grains or greens.

## OSTEOPOROSIS

One woman in two over the age of fifty suffers from *osteoporosis*, characterized by the bones becoming thin, fragile, and easily broken because they no longer contain enough calcium. Scientific studies have shown that there is a greater incidence of osteoporosis in northern Europe and the United States, where dairy and red meat intake is highest, compared with Japan, where very little dairy or red meat is traditionally eaten. Extremely high red meat and dairy consumption causes the calcium to spill into the urine, thus making it unavailable for the body to utilize. Also, as women approach menopause and estrogen production wanes, calcium loss escalates. However, this hormonal-caused depletion of the bones slows after menopause.

### Foods That Promote Bone Loss

Processed foods, carbonated drinks, and red meats contain high amounts of phosphorus, which can deplete the bones. Calcium is more alkaline and helps to balance out phosphorus, which is more acid. Because phosphorus needs to be balanced, the body draws calcium out of the bones.

Excess salt in the diet also produces urine loaded with calcium.[14] Women eating 3900 milligrams sodium daily excreted 30 percent more calcium than those eating 1600 milligrams daily.[15] Avoid processed and canned foods, which contain large amounts of refined salt, and eat sea vegetables, an excellent calcium-rich food, or small amounts of unrefined sea salt instead.

The calcium contained in soybeans can be well absorbed. Studies have shown that subjects who consumed protein entirely from soy excreted about 50 milligrams less urinary calcium than when they consumed equivalent amounts of protein from animal sources.[16]

**Foods that Promote Bone Loss**

Coffee, white sugar, tobacco, alcohol, fiber pills, bran, nutritional yeast, refined salt, processed and canned foods, phosphorus-rich foods, soda pop, white flour, Swiss chard, beet leaves, wood sorrel, rhubarb, cranberries, gooseberries.

*Oxalic acid* is contained in a variety of vegetables and fruits. It can be bound to calcium to form calcium oxalate (solids), which cannot be absorbed, thereby inhibiting calcium absorption. Oxalic acids are found in green leafy vegetables such as Swiss chard, beet leaves, wood sorrel, and spinach, or fruits like rhubarb, cranberries, and gooseberries. For instance, one ounce of cooked spinach will bind 100 to 125 milligrams of its own calcium, making it unavailable for bone nourishment. It is recommended to eat calcium-rich foods when eating foods with oxalic acid.

Green leafy vegetables rich in calcium, such as kale or broccoli, do not contain oxalic acid. In fact, the calcium in these foods is more readily absorbed than the calcium from milk and other dairy products.

Coffee, white sugar, tobacco, alcohol, fiber pills, bran, and nutritional yeast also inhibit calcium absorption or promote calcium excretion, making them undesirable for maintaining bone density. Soaking whole grains, which contain the bran, for at least six to eight hours removes the oxalic acid, making calcium absorption possible.

## Nutrients that Improve Calcium Absorption

Two minerals, boron and magnesium, help maintain calcium balance and prevent postmenopausal calcium loss. Sources of boron and magnesium are apples, pears, apricots, legumes, and nuts. Whole grains, nuts, and pineapples are good sources of manganese, which may also increase calcium absorption.

Vitamin D inhibits calcium loss and promotes calcium absorption. It is important to maintain adequate levels of vitamin D in one's diet or through exposure to the sun. Vitamin D is synthesized in the skin during exposure to ultraviolet rays from the sun. Just ten to fifteen minutes of sunshine a day can help keep your bones strong.

**Nutrients that Improve Calcium Absorption**

Boron, magnesium, manganese, vitamin D, vitamin K, apples, pears, apricots, legumes, nuts, whole grains, pineapples, green leafy vegetables, green tea, kelp, nettles, salmon, halibut, mackerel.

As we age our exposure to the sun is often limited and we tend to use sunscreen, which blocks the UV absorption from sunlight. Elderly women, eighty and older, need at least 600 IU's of vitamin D daily.[17] Fatty fish like salmon, halibut, and mackerel are good sources of vitamin D.

Vitamin K is another essential vitamin to decrease hip fractures. Vitamin K can be found in a variety of foods, such as green leafy vegetables, green tea, kelp, and nettles, and is crucial to calcium absorption.

**Foods Rich in Calcium**

Kukicha tea, herbal infusions, fermented soybeans, lentils, chickpeas, adzuki beans, salmon, sardines, shellfish, collards, bok choy, watercress, kale, broccoli, sesame seeds, tahini, kombu, wakame, nori, dulse, arame, hiziki, sweet potatoes, cabbage, brown rice, millet, barley, whole oats.

| CALCIUM CONTENT OF NATURAL FOODS | |
|---|---|
| **Recommendation for women 50 years old and older is 1200 to 1500 mg of calcium per day.** | |
| Rice: | 1 cup cooked = 25 mg calcium |
| Tofu: | 1 cup = 520 mg calcium |
| Broccoli: | 1 cup cooked = 136 mg calcium |
| Hiziki: | 1 cup cooked = 140 mg calcium |
| Wakame: | 1 cup cooked = 13 mg calcium |
| Kombu: | 1 cup cooked = 8 mg calcium |
| Arame: | 1 cup cooked = 120 mg calcium |
| Chickpeas: | 1 cup cooked = 100 mg calcium |
| Collards: | 1 cup cooked = 300 mg calcium |

# STORIES and PORTRAITS

Charlotte Anderson

Danielle Daniel

Darlene White Eagle

Diane Avoli

Dorothy Golden

# CHARLOTTE ANDERSON

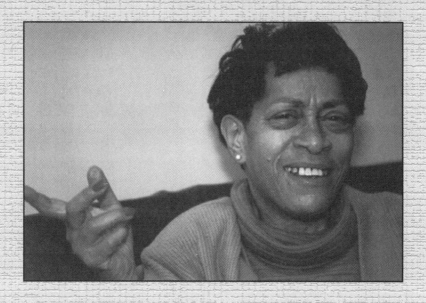

*Ma'* Dear or Big Mom are terms within the African American community that have traditionally been used as terms of endearment, courtesy, reverence, respect, and identification when speaking to the eldest female in the family.

Adult midlife women, in general, were exclusively spoken to and addressed by the titles Mrs. or Miss. These norms were taught early in childhood and strictly adhered to. One knew that these forms of addressing the female within or outside one's immediate family were indicators of the stature and prominence of the woman.

Today, this tradition is more loosely structured. This form of address is no longer taught, practiced, or accepted. Many children are allowed to address the adult female by use of her first name. This is an acceptable practice to the woman being addressed. Children are not taught to pay homage to their female elders anymore.

As a child, I was taught to respond to a question by my female elders with "Yes, Ma'am" or "No, Ma'am" as a sign of respect. In my midlife, I still address my female elders by using these titles. This was common practice, taught and used by children who are today in their forties and fifties.

Women in today's African American culture are more diverse in their thinking, education, and lifestyles than women in their mothers', grandmothers', and great grandmothers' generations. Likewise, the aging process is more diverse than previously. Compared to other cultural groups, African American women age at a less rapid or identifiable rate. It's difficult to determine who is the family matriarch or elder in the community. I hear tales of women who are grandmothers and great grandmothers at thirty or forty years of age. Titles and numbers don't always denote where one is in one's phase of life.

I have grown to accept the aging process. This is a time of freedom from the demands of others. I have raised two children who are independent and live productive lives. I was disconcerted to see my first gray hair in my thirties. This was my first reality check. It no longer troubles me. My daughter, in her late twenties, loves to comb and pat my hair. She says I should apply a rinse to my silver-streaked crown. I laugh, saying, "No, dear, I am perfectly happy to leave my hair as it is. I feel I have earned these stripes. I wear them proudly!"

# DANIELLE DANIEL

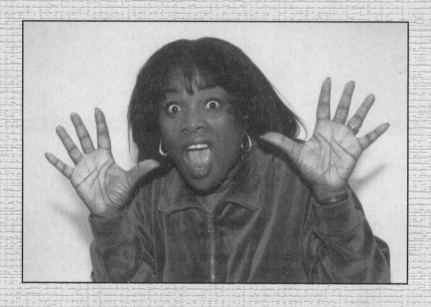

*My* experience of menopause may have been less frightening if I had had more information before it began. I had no idea what was happening when I woke in the middle of the night, sweating profusely. I thought I had eaten something spoiled, but it kept happening every night. My mood changed, and I found myself unattractive and not smart enough anymore. My husband needed to be very understanding. In addition to vaginal dryness I found that my skin and hair were also drier than they used to be. Some lubricants and creams I used were very helpful with these symptoms.

One period, I hemorrhaged for fourteen days. My doctor felt that I was too young, forty-seven at the time, to be going through menopause. Through an ultrasound, he discovered a cyst on my ovary that he believed was causing the problem. I was scheduled for surgery, but my heart would not let me go through with it. The good news is that I have not hemorrhaged since then.

But, I became more depressed and felt as if life was over when my hot flashes got worse. I am a teacher and a performer, and when I got a hot flash while working, I felt that because of my sweating, people thought I was nervous.

There were only a few black women I knew who also went through menopause. Whenever I brought up the subject, most would get quiet. When my sister was diagnosed with cancer and was being treated with chemotherapy, she started having anxiety attacks. The doctor told her she was going through chemically induced menopause. Now, I can pick up the phone and talk to my sister. Before, I felt isolated because I had nobody to relate or share my feelings with.

After reading a book on natural menopause, I started to change my diet. This has helped me immensely. I eliminated dairy, including ice cream. If I eat dairy, I have a hot flash while eating it. Fruits, especially grapes, induce my hot flashes. I eat plenty of vegetables, and chicken and fish, but no red meat.

My whole lifestyle has changed. For instance, I used to enjoy wearing sweaters, but now they cause hot flashes. I have become knowledgeable about herbs for menopause. Though Dong Quai helps some symptoms, I am unable to take it because it can cause a cyst or tumor to grow faster. I need to be careful with other herbs as well. Goldenseal, for instance, would bring on hot flashes.

Now, I no longer have hot flashes; it all depends on the food I eat. The night sweats have stopped, but heat still interferes with my romantic life with my husband. However, I have come to accept the changes, and feel much more in control through self-care and nutrition.

# DARLENE WHITE EAGLE

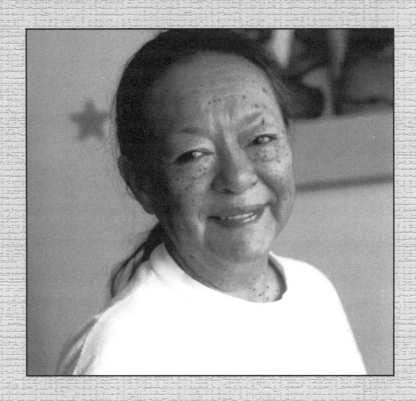

$\mathcal{I}$ was born on the Leech Lake Native American reservation in Minnesota. I have many foster children and foster grandchildren.

There is not much to say about my menopause, because for me it went quickly. I can't even remember the year it happened. What I remember is that I went to a ceremony in South Dakota, and afterwards I had extreme nose bleeding. The next morning I started my monthly cycle. A month later I prepared for another trip, and brought many boxes of napkins, because I did not want to be surprised. But that moon never came.

I did not need estrogen or any other medication women sometimes use when going through menopause. I have heard that because of the changes going on inside, some women leave their families and husbands, get a divorce, or just mysteriously take off. Because I did not feel anything like that, it is hard for me to believe that some women do this.

When I still had my monthly cycle, I had PMS. My emotions reacted to my body symptoms, and I used to get grouchy and cry at the slightest thing. My family knew that it was not because of them that I behaved that way.

Not getting my moon cycle anymore actually makes me happy. Now, I can go to ceremonies or sweat lodges any time. When women are following the traditional Native way of life, they need to learn many valuable tools. One of the teachings is that women need to respect and take care of themselves when they are in their moon. They should not cook or share their food with anyone, nor should they step over anyone or sit on anyone's clothes. They should respectfully keep away from sacred items like tobacco ties, eagle feathers, sacred pipes, and all Native American ceremonies. This is partly because women in their moon contain their own power, which could interfere with the sacred ceremonies.

My advice to women who are having a hard time with the change of life is to learn how to respect, love, and forgive. They should also ask the Creator for help. That is what I do when I need help with my life. Men also need to learn to respect women, because women are here to be honored and to give life. I can only talk about what my own life and culture is all about. But I believe that every woman needs to be in touch with her mind, her body, and her spirit.

DIANE AVOLI

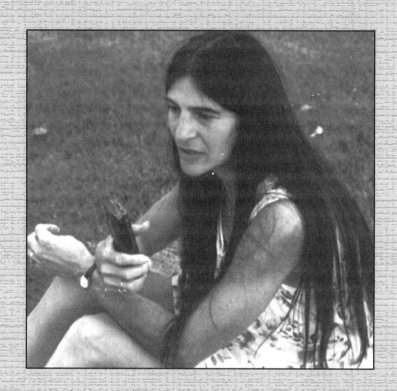

*I* have eight children and one grandchild. My oldest child is twenty-six and my youngest is seven years old.

I started thinking about menopause when my periods were sometimes slightly irregular. In the summer I felt a little bit warm once in a while, although usually heat did not bother me at all. In August I had a perfectly normal menstruation for three days and that was the last one I had. It happened fast for me. It ended and never came back. There was no trickling of the blood and no other symptoms. One day I menstruated and the next day I didn't. In fact, for three months, I kept wondering if I was pregnant. I was even thinking of having a pregnancy test done. My husband said no, and he had always been able to tell.

Since I was in my twenties I have lived a macrobiotic lifestyle. I eat whole grains, beans, land vegetables, and sea vegetables, daily. I think that is the reason I had such a smooth passage into menopause. Because I had no health concerns, I was never on a strict diet. Occasionally, I ate all kinds of foods. But when I had mild flashes of heat, I alleviated them by eating more tofu.

My menopause happened because I had already begun to shift my life. My energies were freed because my youngest child, a seven-year-old boy, did not need me the way the seven girls did. He is very warm and loving and we spend a lot of time together, but he is much more independent. I thought it was interesting that one of my daughters became pregnant right after I went through menopause.

I am still working and developing with my family. But my interests are finally able to extend towards my hobbies of traveling and writing.

Balancing diet and lifestyle can help women ease their passage through menopause. Diet is everything you take in. It is not just the physical food that goes into your mouth. It is your home, your family, your job, everything. Disruptions, stress, too many demands, or unhappiness in your work or relationship, can effect how you experience menopause. In addition to creating harmony and balance within your life situation and adjusting your daily food intake, it is also helpful to just accept what's happening. If you can do that, the menopausal passage can be smooth and positive.

## DOROTHY GOLDEN

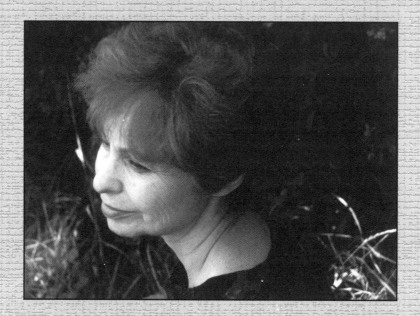

$\mathcal{I}$ have three grown children and Sam, my second husband, has two grown children. I hope to have grandchildren soon.

My signs of menopause were insomnia, tiredness, hot flashes, memory loss, and eyesight loss. I was forty-eight years old at the time. The combination of not sleeping, and being very tired and feeling distressed, made me feel fragile. I was losing my strength inside, which was the worst thing for me.

To combat the symptom of insomnia, I went on Hormone Replacement Therapy. But my breasts became swollen, I gained a lot of weight, and I started bleeding heavily, all of which felt very uncomfortable. In spite of warnings by my doctor, I stopped Hormone Replacement Therapy on my own.

As I was eating a macrobiotic diet for three-and-a-half years, I used more soy products and hoped it would help with my menopausal symptoms. It did help. Although I had been frightened to stop taking hormones, to my surprise the bleeding ceased, and the hot flashes and my other symptoms stopped. The change to eating wisely and going through my passage with natural adjustments helped me to sleep through the night. Other symptoms, like the swelling in my feet and the mucous in my chest, also went away.

I still experience the gradual loss of memory that I hope I can reverse. With new research I believe it will be possible. I also need to work on regaining my sexual desire.

Cookies, breads, and chips, which disrupt my digestive system during this challenging time of menopause, I cut out. Instead of baked goods, I prepare more boiled whole grains and sweet vegetables. I am chewing better and longer and eat less food in general. As a result I have lost my terrible cravings for sweets and lost weight, which makes me feel more sensual.

My general health is better as my body is getting stronger again, like it used to be. Menopause has been more of a tornado than I thought it would be. I am confident that the drawbacks I had during my menopausal journey will subside, and I will continue to follow my newfound path.

# CHAPTER TWO

# BENEFITS of MACROBIOTICS
# for the MENOPAUSAL PASSAGE

We all know that the food we eat and the lifestyle we choose affects our health. Scientific researchers have demonstrated this to us for decades and our own experiences tell us so. Macrobiotics combines these modern research findings with the wisdom of the ages, and offers a way to live and eat in harmony with nature. A way that follows the rhythm of the seasons and the movement of nature's healing forces.

The macrobiotic approach is based on the balance of yin and yang. It uses food and lifestyle that support each other, to realign natural energies and encourage overall well-being. This approach can help women ease their natural cycles with foods that are inherently rich in phytoestrogens, calcium, vitamins, minerals, complex carbohydrates, and proteins.

A balanced macrobiotic lifestyle includes outdoor activities such as gardening, walking, running, or biking. Yoga or other appropriate weight-bearing and stretching exercises should be done on a daily basis, as well as meditation, chanting, or visualization. To relieve menopausal stress, complementary therapies such as homeopathy, aromatherapy, herbal medicine, therapeutic touch, self-massage, shiatsu, acupressure, and acupuncture are excellent methods. They can help one embrace a natural lifestyle and to feel one's best.[18]

In several stories, the women recount the experience of menopause while following a macrobiotic way of life. Some of them lived a natural lifestyle for decades, while others changed their way of life while going through menopause.

Aveline Kushi, who devoted her life to making macrobiotics widely available, encourages whole grains, vegetables, and miso soup, as well as limiting the amount of food one eats while going through menopause.

Shizuko Yamamoto, who brought the Japanese way of massage to the West through her book *Barefoot Shiatsu*, says: "For forty years I have been following a natural macrobiotic lifestyle. I observed that changes occurred slowly over a period of time because macrobiotics embraces a natural healing process. It follows nature's movement, and we are part of that process."

Cecile Tovah Levin, a macrobiotic teacher, reminds us in her story how macrobiotics has helped her, not only with her menopausal passage, but also in her whole life. For her, living in harmony with nature, which includes eating a balanced grain-based diet, was a life worth living.

## WHAT IS MACROBIOTICS?

Macrobiotics is an art and science that is valid and especially useful in today's world. Macrobiotics, a Greek word meaning "great life," refers to living in harmony with nature, eating a simple balanced diet, and living to an active old age. Many philosophers and physicians from all over the world have used the term "macrobiotics" throughout history to signify this. The earliest recorded use of the term "macrobiotics" is found in the writings of Hippocrates.

The beginnings of macrobiotics as we know it today was developed by George Ohsawa from Japan, after he cured himself of a serious illness by adopting a simple diet of brown rice, miso soup, and sea vegetables. Ohsawa integrated Eastern and Western philosophies and medicines to form the dietary and lifestyle principles of what is now known as macrobiotics.

### Contributions to Macrobiotics

During the twentieth century, macrobiotics has influenced people's thinking about nutrition, food as preventive medicine, healing, natural living, and Eastern medicine. We are grateful to George and Lima Ohsawa, Michio and Aveline Kushi, Herman and Cornellia Aihara, and many others, who devoted their lives to teaching macrobiotics.

Macrobiotics is often called "the mother of the natural foods movement." This awareness was sparked in the early sixties, when Michio and Aveline Kushi opened Erewhon, the first natural food store in the United States. The Kushis published numerous books to further the studies of macrobiotics, including *The Book of Macrobiotics: The Universal Way of Health and Happiness* (1977), *Natural Healing* (1978), *The Cancer Prevention Diet* (1983), and *The Complete Guide to Macrobiotic Cooking* (1985).

Macrobiotics acted as a catalyst for the acceptance of alternative and complementary medicine when the Kushi Institute, the premier center for macrobiotic learning, was founded in the late seventies. The Institute now has branches in the United States, Europe, and Japan. The Smithsonian Institution recognized Aveline and Michio Kushi's contributions to the evolution of modern society when it archived documents and artifacts related to their macrobiotic work in the Kushi Family Collection at The National Museum of American History.

### The World of Macrobiotics

Macrobiotics is best known today as a general strengthening and healing diet. The diet emphasizes whole foods, which have been scientifically proven to be beneficial for strong immune systems, high cholesterol reduction, heart disease prevention, weight management, and smoothing menopausal symptoms. Medical professionals often refer their clients to macrobiotics for additional management of certain illnesses.

Many people have given testimonials of how they healed breast cancer, Crohn's disease, and other illnesses with macrobiotic diets, specially designed for them. In 2000, an important study of alternative treatments used by cancer patients reported unconventional treatments, including macrobiotics, effective in reducing stress, minimizing discomforts, and giving patients a sense of control.[19]

However, the majority of people who balance their lifestyle with a macrobiotic approach have no major illness. They do so because it makes them feel good, and it is a great support for a sustainable and peaceful future. Throughout the world, people seeking a holistic and natural approach to physical and spiritual well-being practice macrobiotics.

## The Philosophy

Macrobiotics embraces the Eastern philosophy of Yin and Yang and The Five Energy Transformation Theory. These teachings help us to identify correct daily needs in relation to the food we eat, the people we relate to, and the environment we live in.

Nature is constantly changing through the expanding Yin and contracting Yang forces of the universe. These ever-changing relationships influence our lives, as they are everywhere in nature, and we are part of nature.

The Five Energy Transformation Theory illustrates this constantly changing Yin–Yang relationship in the circle of life, in seasonal as well as in bodily changes. Nature goes through the same stages of growth, development, and death, as we do.

These macrobiotic tools help us adjust to the ever-changing forces of nature, and to live harmoniously. Thus, macrobiotics can help us achieve what we all want: health, peace, happiness, and a long life of prosperity and vitality.

## The Teachings

Macrobiotics teaches awareness for the cycles of nature. As we choose our clothing according to the season, we must learn to choose our food seasonally as well. All foods, including fruits, vegetables, and grains, should be chosen and prepared to balance changes. For instance, in the spring emphasize eating sprouted foods. In winter, implement a longer cooking style, like stews call for. By harmonizing our energy with the environment in this way, we are strengthening body and mind.

To live in harmony with nature means not only eating organic and whole foods, but also using natural fabrics, chemical-free cleaning and gardening products, and organic cosmetics. A natural life supports sustainable businesses and investing, building green buildings, preserving natural living spaces as habitats, and avoiding animal cruelty or testing. Spending time in nature; meditating and reflecting; being helpful, respectful, and grateful for everything, including our ancestors; and giving thanks are all part of the macrobiotic teachings. We must live consciously and responsibly to leave a small imprint on the earth for seven generations to come.

## The Meals

Macrobiotics, with its Eastern philosophical background and its teachers and traditional food items from Japan, is often thought of as a Japanese diet. However, the macrobiotic cuisine has spread its roots into all the traditional diets of the world.

Natural foods are chosen for their strong nutrient and healing properties, and their traditional values. Homemade meals are created with the freshest seasonal and organic ingredients. Whole grains, beans, vegetables, seeds, nuts, sea vegetables, fruits, and oils create a satisfying vegan base for balanced macrobiotic meals. For non-vegan meals, ecologically harvested fish, seafood, or other organic animal products can be prepared. Traditionally fermented foods, such as miso or sauerkraut, provide well-balanced enzymatic seasonings. Foods containing artificial sweeteners, chemical additives, or hormones are not eaten.

Recipes are free of refined foods such as white sugar and flour, and prepared with spring water and non-refined plant or seed oils. A wide variety of cutting and cooking techniques provide an appealing aesthetic at mealtime. Slightly steamed, pressure-cooked, or sautéed, the emphasis is on a variety of tastes and presentations to please the palate and promote balance and health. Raw, sprouted foods and vegetable juices are prepared in the most nutrient saving manners.

Include all food groups when you prepare your meals, to insure adequate nutrition. With all this good food, it is still of utmost importance to chew each mouthful thoroughly, as digestion begins in the mouth. Choose lunch as your main meal. A light meal, eaten three hours before sleep, provides a more restful night.

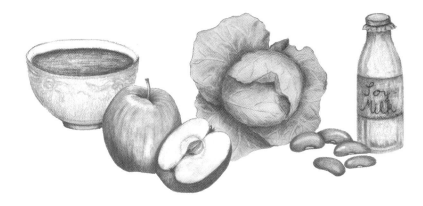

# NATURAL FOOD GUIDELINES

The following macrobiotic natural food guidelines provide a framework for the general use of foods in a temperate climate zone. These guidelines should be individualized depending on gender, age, level of activity, personal needs, and environment. Each menopausal woman must decide which proportions and meal combinations are the best for her needs.

Macrobiotics is about questioning and learning. It is important to study and practice cooking and experience the seasonal changes. To sharpen one's intuition and master the most beneficial selection and preparation of meals, patience and trust in the process is needed.

In the context of disease treatment, during menopause, or if needing detailed guidance in dietary change, one should consult a medical doctor, a nutritionist, and a qualified macrobiotic counselor. The information in this book is not a self-treatment program but a gentle reminder for a balanced and natural lifestyle. It is a re-learning process of the common sense that we have forgotten. When the first step is taken, the natural way of life follows with ease.

## ❀ Animal Foods

Use wild, ocean-ecosystem-friendly fish as well as ecologically farm-raised and harvested fish that are free of contaminants to balance your nutrient intake. Choose white meat fish more often than red meat fish. Monitor the consumption of red meat, poultry, butter, eggs, and all kinds of foods containing dairy. Eat these foods wisely and as needed, and choose only organic products and organic grass-fed meat or wild game. Serve a side dish of grated daikon with a drop of soy sauce with your animal food dishes, to help digestion.

## ❀ Condiments

Condiments enrich the taste and nutrient content of food and can be sprinkled over whole grains or other dishes. Add *gomasio*—a sesame seed and sea salt mixture, *Tekka*—a vegetable miso mixture, or nori or dulse flakes, among others. Many condiments are available ready-made or can be prepared at home. Use them sparingly.

## ❀ Fermented Foods

Complement each meal with a small amount of fermented pickles to enrich your meals with enzymes. Include a pressed or raw salad and sprouted seeds or beans. Prepare homemade quick pickles from a variety of vegetables. Use long-term traditional pickles like raw sauerkraut, *Takuan*—a white radish daikon, or ginger pickles.

## ❀ Fruits

Choose locally grown fruits that are in season to prepare delicious desserts. You can use dried or fresh fruits. Prepare fruits with a pinch of sea salt, or cook them with *kudzu*—a vine with starchy roots. Minimize or avoid eating fruits that cannot be grown in your area.

## ❀ Home Remedies and External Applications

Prepare special combinations of certain foods to eat, drink, or apply externally, for ailments or menopausal symptoms.

## ❀ Land Vegetables

Select daily a variety of vegetable dishes, with an emphasis on green leafy vegetables like collard, kale, broccoli, and nappa cabbage or mustard greens. Select root vegetables like daikon, carrots, burdock, and round vegetables like cabbage, onions, and squash. Choose from many other vegetables within these broad categories. Include small amounts of raw salads, or carrot and green leafy vegetable juices to balance your palate. Minimize nightshades.

## ❀ Legumes, Bean Products, Seeds, and Nuts

Prepare daily dishes made from a variety of beans such as white or black soybeans, chickpeas, adzuki beans, lentils, or traditional bean products like fresh and dried tofu, tempeh, or natto. Soak the beans for eight hours or overnight, and cook them with kombu. Use small amounts of seeds like pumpkin, sesame, sunflower, or flax seeds, and nuts like almonds, chestnuts, or walnuts, and add them to your dishes.

## ❀ Liquids

When thirsty, sip room temperature spring water, Kukicha twigs tea, Bancha tea, green tea, black tea, rice milk, soy milk, or herbal infusion. Strictly avoid carbonated soft drinks. Minimize or avoid coffee, alcohol, and ice cold drinks. Use spring water for all your cooking needs.

## ❀ Oils

Use daily healthy amounts of unrefined oils like first cold-pressed extra virgin olive oil or light sesame oil, and heat them gently. To season salads and other dishes, use a variety of raw oils like walnut oil, toasted sesame oil, extra virgin olive oil or flax seed oil. Minimize deep frying.

## ❀ Seasonings

Mildly flavor dishes with high-quality sea salt, miso, soy sauce, tamari, umeboshi plum vinegar, mirin, sake, wine, rice vinegar, ginger, horseradish, lemon, tangerine, garlic, pepper, or garden herbs. Minimize exotic spices and limit strong salty tastes.

## ❀ Sea Vegetables

Traditionally, many people of the world have cooked with sea vegetables. In the modern towns it is often a forgotten practice, although in the north of France, Maine, Japan, and large parts of Asia, sea vegetables are still harvested and eaten.

Daily, select small amounts of nori, kombu, wakame, dulse, and sweet-water algae to enhance the nutrient content of your meals. Use them as condiments; to accent soups, beans, or vegetable dishes; and prepare larger side dishes—as you would land vegetables—using arame and hiziki, three times per week.

## ❀ Soups

Use daily soups mildly flavored with different kind of traditional fermented miso, tamari, soy sauce, or sea salt, to aid digestion. Include green leafy vegetables, daikon, or carrots and sea vegetables such as wakame and kombu, as well as dried shiitake mushrooms. Use any combination of grains and beans to complement the soups.

## ❀ Supplements

Supplemental enzymes made from whole foods and *probiotics*—naturally occuring bacteria that can improve digestion and health—may be included when digestion slows during the menopausal process. However, adding a daily miso soup and fermented foods to your meals can also remedy this. Herbal tinctures often work well with a natural food lifestyle. Supplements, even when made from food, are often not absorbed, or might not be needed in the amounts the manufacturer recommends them, when eating regularly organic, balanced, natural, and whole meals. However, as with all information in this book, please consult with the appropriate professionals.

## ❀ Sweeteners

Use only natural complex sweeteners like barley malt, brown rice syrup, amazake, or maple syrup. Eat sweet-tasting vegetables like squash, onions, and carrots, or a sweet rice dish. Prepare vegetable juices. Avoid white or brown sugar and sugar substitutes.

## ❀ Whole Grains

Choose un-refined whole grains as the foundation of your natural food lifestyle. A wide variety of whole grains are readily available, like short, long, or medium grain brown rice, sweet rice, red or black rice, wild rice, millet, spelt, barley, oats, hato mugi, kamut, quinoa, wheat, and corn.

Soak the grains overnight or for at least six to eight hours before cooking, which will remove the phytic acid in the bran and make them more digestible. Minimize the intake of whole grain products like flakes, baked flour products like bread (even sour dough), cookies, crackers, and chips. Avoid all man-made products like white or refined flour products, sugars, and starches. Minimize the use of white rice.

# STORIES and PORTRAITS

Lynn Marie Cross

Hannah R. Weinberg

Isabelle Bird Horse

Laurie Savron

Eve Blackwell

LYNN MARIE CROSS

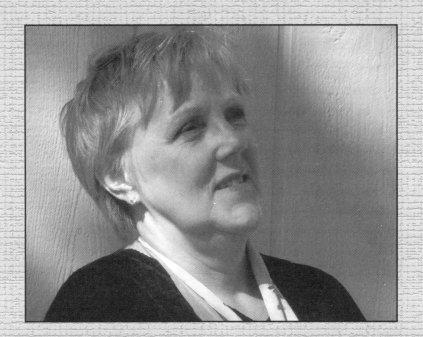

When I was fourteen my periods had not yet begun and I grew impatient. When they finally arrived, they were often very painful and difficult. Yet, their affirmation of fertility and connection with natural, celestial rhythms was reassuring. I gave birth to three lovely daughters. My identity as a woman was found within rhythms of fertility. It was all I knew of life, and I did not want to imagine life without it.

When I was forty-eight, the first signs of menopause appeared with less-regular intervals between menses. Though I knew the transition was as natural as menarche, this time I was not eager. I grieved for the loss of the Mother. Sometimes this feeling actually overshadowed the unpleasantness of hot flashes.

The physical symptoms were not extreme or intolerable. I think perhaps my macrobiotic diet of lots of tofu, tempeh, and other soy products, which are thought to be useful in maintaining hormone levels, helped. Maintaining an overall balance on a daily basis, with grains and vegetables as my dietary mainstays, made the wild swings that are so typical of this time of life softer.

Wild yam cream, topically applied, to moderate hot flashes; yellow dock tincture to support my liver and digestive tract; and black cohosh tincture, I used for additional balancing. I practiced yoga, walked outdoors daily, and did strength training. I am sure that all of these things kept my hormones on an even keel, without resorting to HRT supplementation.

The emotional impact was another matter. I felt adrift, cut off from productive life. Many other uprooting life changes occurred around my fiftieth year. My marriage dissolved, I left my house, I lost my job, and my children began to leave the nest. I had gained weight and felt unattractive. Is THIS menopause? I asked. When things fall apart? At the lowest point, I said NO! This is not the way to live!

I am eagerly learning new things and developing new job skills. My creative life has begun to show a new richness. I am beginning to understand that my connection with life's rhythms has not been severed at all. I see this midlife transition as part of an even larger rhythm. It feels like a birth, or an entrance into a new country. Yet it's not unfamiliar. I am coming home to myself, and a lifetime of discovery lies ahead.

Friends and children are wonderfully supportive. My women friends, particularly those who perform with me in the Wild Yam Cabaret, help me laugh, which is so essential to keeping one's head on straight. The girls at one time fought me in my attempts to keep their diets in macrobiotic balance. Now they have matured into understanding and gratefully use the principles, which I hoped they were somehow absorbing. They are a great source of joy and continued discovery.

As I approach the close of my menopausal passage, I see the need for an inward focus. It is a time to step back, to take stock, and plant new seeds. It is not about decline, but about assembling the pieces in a new way.

HANNAH R. WEINBERG

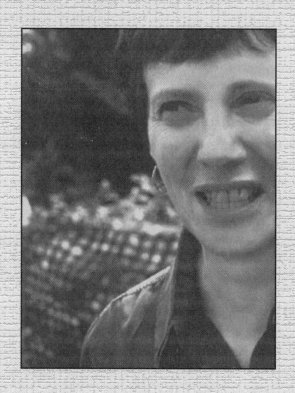

*I* have two grown children and three grandchildren.

The changes in my menstrual cycle started in the summer when I had periods about two weeks apart. The next summer, the same thing happened, but more frequently. My gynecologist did an endometrial biopsy to rule out problems due to bleeding. At that time she advised me to take estrogen replacement, to regulate my periods. I decided against it, to see how I would do on my own.

Over the next several years, I started to experience more irregularities, some hot flashes at night, and insomnia. I woke up every night around four o'clock, and had problems falling back to sleep. This lasted for three years till I stopped having periods in my early fifties.

Now, I am free of all symptoms and feel well. I am not taking any Hormone Replacement Therapy. However, I have adopted a macrobiotic diet and eat foods rich in phytoestrogens, like the soybean products of tofu and miso. To combat osteoporosis, I exercise three times a week, including weight lifting, aerobics, and yoga. By avoiding animal fats, I hope to minimize or eliminate osteoporosis and prevent heart problems, some of the frightening consequences of aging. My relationship with my husband is better than ever. A postmenopausal woman does not have to worry about pregnancy, and this has been liberating for us.

When my menopausal symptoms started, it was difficult to consider natural menopause. It seems that most doctors, many of my friends, and society in general expect a woman to take hormones. Fortunately, my doctor, who is female and also postmenopausal, respected my wishes. She herself takes HRT in order to keep her mind "sharp." She asked me if I had any problems in that regard, but I did not think so.

As a woman in midlife I try to reduce stress through meditation and yoga. Having friends to talk to, a good diet and regular exercise, meaningful work and a good relationship, helped me through this stage of life. Looking at this list, however, everyone at any age would benefit from these things.

It is very important to stay busy after menopause. I run a small business in the scientific field, and although challenging, it allows me to be creative in my own way. Hopefully, I will find new creative outlets when I retire from this work.

## ISABELLE BIRD HORSE

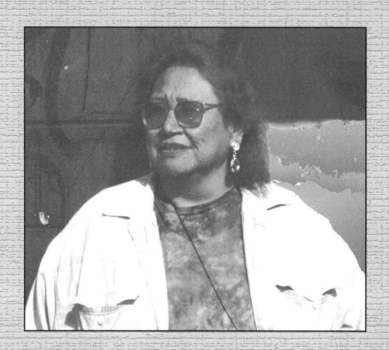

*I* was born at Standing Rock Sioux Reservation in Fort Yates, North Dakota. The oldest of ten children, I have nine children of my own.

I don't remember my grandmother talking about menopause. Maybe she thought it wasn't time for her to tell me. When my mother went through menopause in her mid-fifties she never explained it to me either. I only remember my grandmother telling me how to become a woman and what an honor it was to bring children into the world. She talked about our relation to Mother Earth, and the four phases of our lives in relation to the four seasons of the year. Spring and summer is the time of birth and growing up. Fall and winter is the period of old age and the dying time.

When I was forty-one years old I had my last child through Caesarian section and had my tubes tied. At the time I was in such pain, I didn't care. A year later I regretted my decision, because I felt I had lost my worth. I thought, "What good am I now, that I can't bear children?" I realized that I was getting old. I felt dried up, like an old crone. My interest in sex wasn't there. It's still not there. I had hot flashes, dizzy spells, and emotional turmoil. Yet, I did nothing to alleviate the pain. I was grieving. It was like I was dying in my mind. It was a slow death. Being diabetic is stressful enough, but going through artificially induced menopause in addition felt overwhelming.

After surgery I had a spiritual turnover. I started relying on the Great Spirit and learned to walk the Red Road. Walking the Red Road meant that I started each day with prayers and continued through the day. By communicating with my inner spirit and learning to be with my spirit, I let go of many things and coped better with ups and downs. Without prayers through my menopause I wouldn't have had harmony or inner strength.

I see a lot of women from different cultures. Some don't talk about their issues, but manifest them in physical illnesses. I think we all need to share and talk about our lives. Life is one big circle and we are all connected. If we don't share and teach others about our lives, then the journey, our circle, gets broken, and we have a hard time trying to mend that break. Life can be very stressful if we are not there to support each other.

# LAURIE SAVRAN

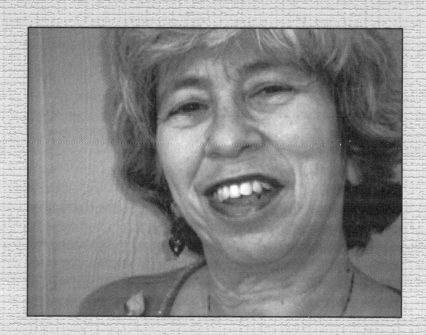

$\mathscr{I}$ am the mother of two daughters and I have two grandchildren.

When I was in my forties, I saw a gynecologist because I had missed my period for several months. He told me I might menstruate again because the color of my uterus still looked pink. He warned that when it is all over the color is darker and less vibrant. Still, I cried grief-filled tears of disbelief, because I had thought that I would go through menopause in my fifties.

Periods were not a problem for me. I had been a late bloomer, with my first period at sixteen when I looked like a child of twelve. I never experienced cramping or pre-menstrual stress and my two pregnancies were normal. I am not late this time, but early, an unprecedented physiological experience for me. I have missed three periods in the past eighteen months, and have had hot flashes for six months. The hot flashes are actually pleasurable, as most of the time I am cold.

But, I'm not ready for this yet. It all happened too fast. Men don't notice me on the streets since I let my hair go gray. I don't mind a lot, but I do mind. Men are inherently attracted to someone who can fulfill their need to procreate. I can't provide that anymore. Does it mean I'm losing my femininity and charms as a woman?

On the other side, menopause, with its horror stories of depression, hot flashes, and osteoporosis, has been easy for me. I guess I should feel relieved and grateful. Nature is being gentle to me, and the choice of having more children is not a concern anymore. But, is dying coming sooner than I thought as well? I remember the wrinkles on my mother's neck. Have they been passed on to me? Will I be more susceptible to cancer of the breast? All these questions well up inside me where the mystery happens. The red blood will not flow for me again; the sacrifice to Mother Earth is already made.

Menopause was a time of transformation, physiologically, emotionally, and spiritually. During my menstrual years, I grew slowly, healing the past and raising my family. I analyzed my family of origin and worked to understand the dysfunctional aspects of my relationship with my parents.

When menopause came, it was time to grow up. There was the duty to forgive the past and create my future, and to be responsible for fulfilling my dreams. My children were analyzing and criticizing me, and I knew without a doubt that relying on appearances wasn't the answer. I also understood that my self-worth had to come from inside me.

In Buddhism, the Wheel of Life is the mundane world. The goal is to get off the wheel into nirvana. Menopause gets you off one kind of wheel. Why not view it as a path to enlightenment? Menopause is the time of ultimate freedom in a woman's life. But she must make the choice to be free.

EVE BLACKWELL

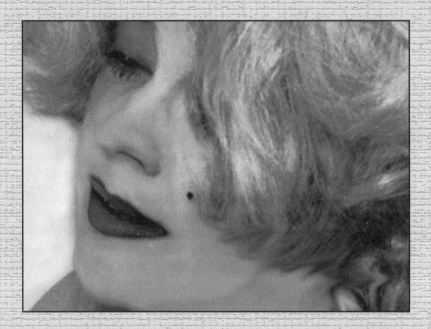

$\mathcal{S}$ome years ago, LIFE magazine celebrated half a century of publishing. On its cover were tiny replicas of over five hundred feature photos in a collage that made a startling composite: the face of Marilyn Monroe.

Why was this tragic icon chosen to symbolize the collective identity of our culture? Cynics might sum it up in two words: "Marilyn sells." But, why does she sell? What does she sell? Why haven't we let her go? And what does this have to do with a middle-aged writer, performer, and grandmother like me?

As an adolescent in the fifties, I hated "MM," as the promotions billed her. In those days girls were good or bad. The latter were like Marilyn, in tight skirts and sweaters, openly French-kissing around the corner from the principal's office. To emulate them was to be ostracized, criticized, and seen as intriguing and scary. Marilyn's baby voice, low necklines and exaggerated wiggles made us "good girls" feel vulnerable and ashamed of being female. Though some of us stuffed Kleenex into our bras and fantasized about fooling around in cars, we didn't talk about it.

In the sixties we marched for freedom, joined co-ops, and baked organic bread. Few of us read Marilyn's posthumously published "autobiography," which had been rewritten by three men.

In the seventies we read Betty Friedan, Gloria Steinem, and Germaine Greer. These were educated white women who challenged us to expand traditional roles. We may have forgotten to listen to our sisters of color or of different economic and educational backgrounds. We also forgot about Marilyn. She was dead, probably a circumstance triggered by low self-esteem; too uncomfortable to think about.

By the eighties Marilyn's ripe body seemed "kitsch." Women were all jogging and dieting to look "lean and mean" in business suits. Who cared about tight dresses with breasts and belly bursting out?

When I reached middle age, my opinion of Marilyn had not changed. Her image stared at me from posters, magazines, and pop art. A reminder of what I would never want to be. My own body was changing. I had a hysterectomy, along with half the women of my generation. Somehow, the removal of the huge fibroid helped me to push out the fear and self-loathing I had accumulated in my life and begin to birth my creative voice.

The Muse sent me Marilyn. I was shocked, frightened, appalled. What could Marilyn have to do with my artistic process? She was not my type. I clung to the memory of my master's thesis on Shakespeare's heroines that lay mildewing in the basement of my university's library. I remembered the feminist books and women's groups I had attended so earnestly. What on earth would my friends think?

But the Muse would not be denied. I bought a blond wig and stuffed myself into a dress that made me feel like a sausage sprayed in gold lame. Then I went to work coaxing my middle-aged body to move in a way that, by current standards, I knew was politically incorrect.

To dare to be the Love Goddess at fifty-one! Now, when my chin, waist, and belly had expanded with the fullness of my years! What would it be like? I soon found out.

Audience response was all over the map. Some folded their arms and shook their heads. Others giggled and smiled as if they had taken catnip. One man, from the World War II generation, attended most performances because he "just liked Marilyn." Women—young and old alike—said, "Marilyn brought up a curious pain" and "I didn't know whether to laugh or cry." A reviewer said he'd heard it all before.

Two audiences stopped the show with applause. My body took it all in, trembling uncontrollably before stepping on stage, sobbing in the bathroom before the very first show. I moved from one line to the next, aware that they invited comparisons in a world that worshiped the young and famous.

On the other side of the process was freedom. I have stopped caring what people think. As Marilyn's dress has constricted my body, writing in her voice has expanded my mind. Her screen persona had been a cleverly devised clown, the wise child within the woman. Like the goddess Aphrodite, she mirrored back one's projections. Walking in her three-inch heels, I began to see that her softness and receptivity went hand-in-hand with her shrewdness. She directed her career with the cunning of a brigadier general.

I stopped judging Marilyn. I began to settle into my softness and vulnerability and see them as strengths. I said what I thought and let my temper fly when I felt like it. Marilyn now felt like a sister, who had struggled to define herself in a world that minimized values we define as "feminine."

What are those values? Building human spirit, nurturing families and communities, connecting with the earth, and honoring process as well as product, these are some. We who can house new life and nurture it within our bodies are intimately acquainted with the creative process, with sharing and living in community. Our wisdom, our art, our ideas are needed in the great healing that challenges us locally, nationally, and globally.

It is the fear of judgment that keeps most people from the fullest expression of their creativity. For women, part of that expression is in our stories, our songs, our art, our quilts, and our crafts. Let's get them all out of the closets, attics, and drawers. If life isn't a cabaret, it is at least a playground, where no one child's opinion counts more than another's.

If Marilyn's life was a parable, perhaps we had better look closer. Her real message may not have been about whom she slept with or whether she was murdered. Maybe the message was about our idea of woman as a victim, or our refusal to accept that vulnerability comes with the capacity for strength. With this strength comes the responsibility to embrace our pain and speak from it in whatever way we can. To help each other up the mountain and to see the whole world as family.

There is a great mystery in the feminine spirit. In your story and mine is the mystery of the feminine in all of us that cries for expression and balance in the world. That mystery gave us the child, woman, artist, sex goddess, and the fierce opportunist that was Marilyn Monroe. In a sense, we are all those things, and so we are all Marilyn. Perhaps that is why we have not let her go.

# CHAPTER THREE
# NATURAL FOOD RECIPES

A balanced natural food lifestyle is an essential tool to support the menopausal passage. With the understanding that phytoestrogens are available in whole foods, we should increase their intake during the midlife years.

The following recipes are divided into nine sections—whole grains, soups, beans, vegetable dishes, salads, dressings, fermented foods, fish recipes, and desserts. The recipes include menu suggestions and list variations of different ingredients and cooking methods to inspire new creations with minimal effort. Each dish serves about four to seven people, depending on the portion size and what you serve with the dish.

## WHOLE GRAINS

# BREAKFAST PORRIDGE

Serves 4

*This is a nourishing breakfast porridge that can be eaten year round. You can use a mixture of different grains, or just brown rice, or any other grain alone. Use leftover grain from dinner, or make a fresh batch using the Brown Rice recipe on page 67.*

| |
|---|
| 2 cups cooked whole grain of your choice |
| 5 cups spring water |
| Dulse flakes |

**Preparation:** Combine cooked grain with water. Stir, and bring to a boil. Cover the pot and simmer for about 20 minutes. For a creamier texture, use a blender. Serve hot and garnish with dulse flakes, a sea vegetable.

**Variation:** You can season the porridge with miso or gomasio, or use rice syrup for a sweet taste. Try cooking the grain with rice or soy milk instead of water. Add seasonal fruits or vegetables while cooking the grain.

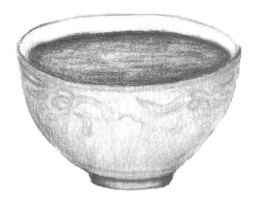

# BROWN RICE

Serves 4 to 7

*Cultivated throughout the world, rice is a universal food. Brown rice is the most nourishing grain, and possibly the most delicious. Its naturally sweet taste can be enjoyed on a daily basis. For a complete meal, eat the rice with a bean dish, a variety of vegetables, fermented pickles, and gomasio. Serve with a miso soup. (See page 71 for recipe.)*

| |
|---|
| 2 cups organic short grain brown rice |
| 3 cups spring water, for pressure cooking |
| 4 cups spring water, for boiling |
| Pinch of sea salt, per cup of rice |
| Parsley, finely chopped for garnish |

**Preparation:** *Pressure cooking* ~ Clean 2 cups of organic short grain brown rice, add 3 cups of spring water, and briefly heat. Soak overnight with a few drops of rice vinegar. The next day, discard soaking water and replace with 3 cups of fresh spring water and 1 pinch of sea salt per cup of rice. Place rice and water in the pressure cooker and start to boil the water on medium high. When the water boils, add the sea salt and fasten down the cover. When the pressure is up, reduce the flame to medium low and place a metal flame deflector under the pressure cooker. Pressure cook the rice for 45 to 50 minutes. Remove the pot and let the pressure completely down. Take off the cover and allow the rice to sit for 4 minutes. Mix the rice and scoop it into a wooden bowl.

*Boiling* ~ Clean 2 cups of organic short grain brown rice, add 4 cups of spring water, and briefly heat. Soak overnight with a few drops of rice vinegar. The next day, discard the soaking water; replace with 3 cups of spring water and 1 pinch of sea salt per cup of rice. Bring to a boil. Cover the pot, place a flame deflector under the pot, and let it simmer on low heat for 45 to 50 minutes. Let the rice rest in the pot for 4 minutes. Mix the rice and place it in a wooden bowl and serve.

**Variation:** Choose from a variety of rice including short, medium, long, sweet, black, red, and basmati rice. Prepare combination dishes by adding $1/4$ cup of other soaked whole grains like barley, millet, or wild rice, or a variety of beans like black soybeans, lentils, or chickpeas, and cook it with your choice of rice. Use brown rice as a base for a variety of dishes like rice salad, fried rice, rice soup, rice balls, or sushi rolls.

# MILLET a la MASHED POTATO

Serves 4

*Millet is a staple grain in Africa. In Ethiopia, the black millet is only used to make local beer, the red is prepared as pita bread, and the white millet is mainly for Injera—soft, fluffy sourdough bread. Use millet as a main dish with vegetables, beans, and miso soup, or as a breakfast grain. The cauliflower is a substitute for the texture and taste of the potato.*

| |
|---|
| 1 cup millet, clean |
| 2 cups cauliflower, cut into bite-size pieces |
| 3–4 cups spring water |
| Pinch of sea salt |
| Sesame seeds, slightly toasted |

**Preparation:** Clean 1 cup of millet and add 3 to 4 cups of spring water. Briefly heat. Add a few drops of rice vinegar and soak overnight. The next day, discard soaking water and replace it with 3 to 4 cups of spring water. Then place the millet, cauliflower, water, and a pinch of salt in a pot and bring to a boil. Lower heat and simmer for about 30 minutes. Remove and serve with toasted sesame seeds as garnish.

**Variation:** Roast the millet for a nutty flavor, or pressure cook the dish. Add garlic, onions, or squash for a different taste.

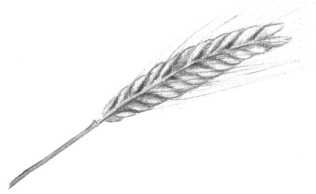

# NOODLE SALAD

Serves 3 to 4

*Noodles are delicious and more easily digestible than baked flour products. Noodles can be eaten as a snack alone, or served with vegetables and a tofu side dish as a meal.*

| |
|---|
| 1 pack udon whole wheat noodles |
| 3 quarts spring water |
| 3 tablespoons soy sauce, to taste |
| 1 tablespoon ginger juice, to taste |
| 2 sprigs of scallions, finely cut |
| $^1/_2$ tablespoon dulse flakes |

**Preparation:** Bring water to a boil. Add the noodles and boil for about 10 minutes while adding additional small amounts of cold water. Drain and rinse quickly. Add scallions, soy sauce, ginger juice, and dulse to the noodles, and mix.

**Variation:** Use soba buckwheat noodles or rice noodles. Serve the noodles in a broth. Prepare the broth by adding a 2-inch long piece of kombu and one shiitake mushroom to 3 cups of water and boil for 10 minutes. Season with soy sauce and ginger juice to taste and serve with noodles of your choice. Garnish with finely cut scallions and nori flakes.

# WILD RICE DISH

Serves 3

*Wild rice grown by Northern tribes in Minnesota is my favorite. It is still harvested in their traditional way and served with walleye, corn, and blueberries.*

| |
|---|
| 1 cup wild rice |
| 2 cups spring water or vegetable broth |
| Pinch of sea salt |
| 1 cup mushrooms |
| 1 tablespoon extra virgin olive oil |

**Preparation:** Clean 1 cup of wild rice and add 2 cups of spring water. Briefly heat. Add a few drops of rice vinegar and soak overnight. The next day, discard soaking water and replace it with 2 cups of either spring water or vegetable broth. Add a pinch of sea salt and bring to a boil. Simmer on a low flame for about 30 to 35 minutes. Fluff the cooked rice with a fork. Meanwhile, sauté the mushrooms in olive oil until brown. Combine the wild rice with the mushrooms and serve hot.

**Variation:** Wild rice is great in casseroles or in soups. Cook it together with Brown Rice. (See page 67 for recipe.)

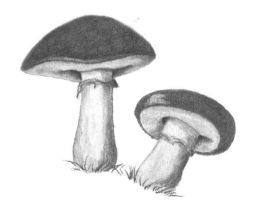

# SOUPS

MISO SOUP
VEGETABLE STEW
SWEET CORN SOUP
LENTIL SOUP with DANDELION

*Soups*

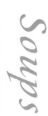

# MISO SOUP

Serves 4

*Miso is a fermented bean paste that provides a wide variety of enzymes and bacteria, which are beneficial to the digestive system and aid in food absorption. It also contains proteins, vitamins, and minerals. Add miso to a variety of other soups and dishes for seasoning.*

| |
|---|
| 4 cups spring water |
| 1 dried shiitake mushroom |
| 1 cup daikon |
| $1/4$ cup onions |
| 2 tablespoons wakame (sea vegetable) |
| $1/4$ pound tofu |
| 5–6 teaspoons of barley miso |
| Scallions, finely sliced for garnish |

**Preparation:** To begin, soak the shiitake mushroom for 10 minutes and slice; dice the onions very small; slice the diakon into thin quarter moons; soak the wakame for 5 minutes and slice; and puree the barley miso with a small amount of warm water. Next, bring the water to a boil. Add the wakame and shiitake mushrooms and simmer for 5 minutes. Then add the vegetables and tofu and simmer for another 5 minutes. Next, mix the miso puree into the soup and gently simmer for 3 to 5 minutes, being careful not to boil the soup. Serve hot and garnish with scallions.

**Variation:** Use any combination of vegetables. Add cooked grains like barley or beans like lentils to the soup. Choose different flavors of miso like barley, rice, soybean, mellow rice, or chickpea. Garnish with parsley.

# VEGETABLE STEW

Serves 4 to 6

*This vegetable stew is very nourishing because it is loaded with minerals, especially calcium, and rich in vitamins and protein. It can be served with a piece of whole grain sourdough bread or with a grain and vegetable dish.*

| |
|---|
| 1 tablespoon extra virgin olive oil |
| 1 cup onions |
| 4–6 cups vegetable broth or spring water |
| 1 cup mushrooms |
| 2 cups root vegetables, carrots, parsnip, and burdock |
| 1 cup winter squash |
| 1 lb tofu |
| $^1/_4$ cup of wakame sea vegetable, soaked for 5 minutes, cut small |
| **SEASONING** |
| 5 teaspoons miso paste, pureed with a small amount of warm water |
| 1 teaspoon umeboshi plum vinegar, optional |
| $^1/_4$ cup tahini sesame butter |
| Parsley, finely chopped for garnish |

**Preparation:** First cube the tofu, winter squash, carrots, parsnip, and burdock. Clean and quarter the mushrooms and chop the onions. Soak the wakame for 5 minutes and then cut small. Then, sauté first the onions, then the mushrooms, the root vegetables, and the winter squash in olive oil. Add vegetable broth or water and cook for 20 minutes, or until the vegetables are tender. Towards the end, gently place the tofu, the wakame, and the seasoning into the stew and continue to simmer on a low flame for 5 to 7 minutes. Garnish with parsley.

**Variation:** You can add cabbage, Brussels sprouts, and turnips, or any other variation of vegetables, including grains or beans, to the stew. For a thick consistency add 1 to 2 tablespoons of kudzu dissolved in 4 tablespoons of cold water and stir until it thickens.

# SWEET CORN SOUP

Serves 4 to 6

*This is a delicious and sweet soup to enjoy in the summer season.*

| |
|---|
| 4 ears of corn |
| 1 large onion |
| 2 carrots |
| 2 stalks of celery |
| Nori sea vegetable |
| 1 teaspoon light sesame oil |
| 4 teaspoons mellow rice miso, diluted with warm water |
| 4–6 cups of spring water |

**Preparation:** Begin by dicing the onion, carrots, and celery. Remove the kernels from the corn. Sauté the onions in sesame oil until translucent. Add carrots, celery, and corn, then the water, and bring to a boil. Reduce heat and simmer for about 15 to 30 minutes, or until vegetables are soft. Add miso to the soup and simmer for five minutes. Garnish with nori strips that have been toasted and cut into thin strips, and serve.

**Variation:** Adding another vegetable or omitting one will vary the taste of the soup. Puréeing the soup in a blender or eating it cold is another option. You can also roast the corn before adding it to the soup. Use fresh or frozen corn.

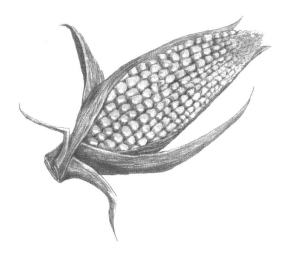

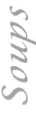
# LENTIL SOUP with DANDELION

Serves 4 to 6

*Preparing lentils with dandelion and umeboshi vinegar adds a sour-bitter touch to the dish, which improves digestion. Dandelion strengthens the liver.*

| |
|---|
| 1 cup French lentils |
| ¹/₂ cup onions |
| ¹/₂ cup carrots |
| ¹/₄ cup celery |
| 1 small piece of kombu sea vegetable |
| 1 bunch of dandelion |
| 4–6 cups spring water |
| 2 tablespoons of tamari or soy sauce, to taste |
| 2 teaspoons umeboshi plum vinegar or apple cider vinegar, to taste |
| Scallions, sliced for garnish |

**Preparation:** Wash and soak the lentils for a few hours. Dice the celery and onions; cube the carrots; wash and cut very fine the dandelion; and soak kombu in spring water for 5 minutes. Place the kombu at the bottom of the pot, then add the onions, carrots, and lentils. Add the spring water, bring to a boil, and simmer for about 30 minutes. Remove the cooked kombu, add dandelion, and continue simmering on a low flame until the greens are soft. Add tamari and umeboshi plum vinegar to the soup and simmer for 5 minutes. Garnish with chopped scallions or parsley.

**Variation:** You can add any kind of greens to this soup, like broccoli, chives, kale, or collards. Use other beans like chickpeas or green, brown, or yellow lentils. Season with different kinds of miso flavors.

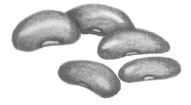

# BEANS

ADZUKI BEANS with SQUASH
TEMPEH SALAD
PAN-FRIED TOFU
PAN-FRIED TOFU IN KUDZU SAUCE
SCRAMBLED TOFU

*Beans*

# ADZUKI BEANS with SQUASH

Serves 4 to 7

*Adzuki are small, compact, shiny red beans that are lower in fat and oil than other beans. Adzuki beans strengthen the kidneys and, cooked with squash, give nourishment to the spleen as well.*

| |
|---|
| 1 cup adzuki beans |
| 2–3 cups buttercup squash |
| 3–6 inch long strip of kombu seaweed |
| 2–3 cups spring water |
| $1/4$ teaspoon sea salt, per cup of beans |
| Scallions, minced for garnish |

**Preparation:** Wash 1 cup of adzuki beans and add 2 to 3 cups of spring water. Briefly heat. Add a few drops of lemon and soak overnight. The next day, discard soaking water and replace it with 2 to 3 cups of spring water. Cut the squash into large 1-inch chunks; soak the kombu seaweed for five minutes. Then place the adzuki beans with the kombu and squash in a pressure cooker. Add enough spring water to cover the squash chunks and fasten the cover. Turn the flame to high and bring to pressure. When you hear the hissing sound, reduce the flame to medium low and place a flame deflector under the pressure cooker. Cook for 45 to 50 minutes. Bring the pressure down completely. Remove the cover and season with sea salt and mix gently. Simmer for about 15 minutes. Place the beans and squash in a serving bowl and garnish with scallions.

**Variation:** Boil the beans for 2 hours while gently adding cold water. For a different taste, add miso or soy sauce to season after the beans are soft. Adzuki beans can also be eaten plain or cooked with brown rice or wheat berries. When sweetened with barley malt or cooked with dried chestnuts, adzuki beans make a delicious dessert. Use Hokkaido pumpkin or butternut squash.

# TEMPEH SALAD

Serves 4 to 5

*Tempeh is a whole fermented soybean product that is traditionally eaten in Indonesia. This chewy, satisfying, and easily digested soy food provides great energy and restores vitality. It is rich in protein and many other important nutrients, and can be prepared in a variety of delicious ways.*

| |
|---|
| 8 ounces of tempeh |
| Stamp-size kombu |
| Spring water, enough to cover tempeh |
| 2 tablespoons soy sauce, or to taste |
| 4–6 kosher cucumber pickles |
| 2 stems of broccoli florets |
| 1 cup onion |
| 4 sprigs scallions |
| 2 tablespoons light sesame oil |
| Parsley, chopped for garnish |
| **DRESSING** |
| 2 teaspoons Dijon mustard, diluted with 5–7 tablespoons cold water |
| 1–2 tablespoons umeboshi plum vinegar, to taste |
| 1–2 tablespoons soy sauce, to taste, or salt |
| 2 tablespoons extra virgin olive oil |
| $1/2$ tablespoon of dulse flakes |

**Preparation:** Cube the tempeh and cucumber pickles; dice the onion and the scallions; clean and soak the kombu; and cut the broccoli florets into small pieces. Then, on the stove, heat the sesame oil. Add and gently toss the tempeh until golden brown on all sides. Remove the tempeh and place on a paper napkin for 5 minutes to remove excess oil. Place tempeh and kombu into a pot and cover with spring water. Add the soy sauce and bring to a boil, then simmer for 20 minutes. In a separate pot, boil the broccoli until crunchy, remove, and do the same with the onions. Mix the dressing with a whisk or fork. Combine the tempeh, broccoli, onions, scallions, cucumber pickles, and dressing, and then lightly toss. Let marinate for a while and serve with fresh parsley for garnish.

**Variation:** Tempeh can be added to many dishes and soups, and also makes a great sandwich combined with lettuce, sprouts, and a spread on naturally fermented sourdough bread.

# PAN-FRIED TOFU

Serves 4

*Tofu is a high-protein food made from soybeans and is easy to digest. It is prepared by carefully removing the crude fiber and water-soluble carbohydrats from white soybeans. Tofu is low in saturated fats and cholesterol, and rich in minerals and vitamins. A good source of phytoestrogens, tofu can be eaten more often during the midlife transition. Pan-Fried Tofu is a great snack as is, or can be eaten with a sourdough sandwich with lettuce and sprouts.*

| |
|---|
| 1 pound firm tofu |
| 2–3 tablespoons light sesame oil or olive oil |
| 2 tablespoons soy sauce, to taste |

**Preparation:** Press tofu with a heavy weight for a half hour. Then towel dry and cut into even slices. Gently heat oil in a heavy skillet and place the dried tofu slices in the pan. Gently fry the tofu on both sides until brown, adding more oil if needed. Use a protection screen to avoid the splashing of oil. Remove the browned tofu and put on several paper towels to absorb the excess oil. At this point, the tofu can be marinated with a few tablespoons of soy sauce or boiled in a water-and-soy sauce mixture for 5 minutes.

**Variation:** See recipe on the next page.

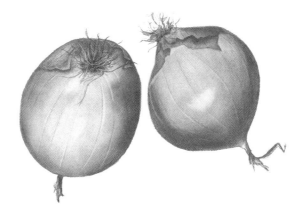

# PAN-FRIED TOFU in KUDZU SAUCE

Serves 4

*Pan-Fried Tofu in Kudzu Sauce is my favorite tofu dish. Serve it with Millet a la Mashed Potatoes (page 68) and green leafy vegetables.*

| |
|---|
| 1 pound firm tofu |
| 2–3 tablespoons light sesame oil or olive oil |
| 1–2 tablespoons kudzu |
| 1 cup of onions |
| 1 cup of carrots |
| 2–4 cups spring water |
| 3 tablespoons of soy sauce, to taste |
| Ginger juice, to taste |
| Parsley, minced for garnish |

**Preparation:** Press tofu with a heavy weight for a half hour. Then towel dry and cut into 8 even slices. Dilute the kudzu with a small amount of cold water, and cut the onions and carrots into small cubes. Gently heat oil in a heavy skillet and place the towel-dried tofu slices in the pan. Gently fry the tofu on both sides until brown, adding more oil if needed. Remove the browned tofu and put on several paper towels to absorb the excess oil. After the excess oil is absorbed, place the tofu in a pot on top of the onions and carrots. Add a little more spring water than it takes to cover the tofu, carrots, and onions, and about 3 tablespoons of soy sauce, or to taste. Bring to a boil, and then simmer for 15 to 20 minutes. Pour the diluted kudzu liquid into the simmering water and stir continuously, until the white color of the kudzu becomes clear and the water thickens. Season again with soy sauce and add ginger juice to taste. Garnish with parsley and serve hot.

# SCRAMBLED TOFU

Serves 3 to 4

*Scrambled Tofu is an easy-to-digest breakfast dish that resembles scrambled eggs. It is delicious and satisfies the need for phytoestrogens. It can also be served as a bean protein side dish with lunch or dinner.*

| |
|---|
| 1 pound soft tofu |
| 2 tablespoons extra virgin olive oil |
| 3 scallions |
| 2–3 tablespoons soy sauce |
| $1/2$ sheet nori, cut into small pieces |
| Parsley, minced for garnish |

**Preparation:** Press tofu with a heavy weight for a half hour, then towel dry. Cut the nori into small pieces. Cut all parts of the scallions into thin slices. Heat oil in a pan. Break tofu into small pieces with your hand, and place them into the pan. Sauté for several minutes until browned, stir, and continue sautéing. Add the scallions, the soy sauce, and a little bit of water. Simmer on a low flame for about 5 minutes. Mix in the nori pieces. Garnish with parsley and serve hot.

**Variation:** Use different vegetables, like broccoli, celery, parsley, or carrots, or use a mixture of vegetables. Experiment with seasonings like salt, black pepper, tumeric, garlic, ginger, or curry powder in your scrambled tofu. Instead of nori, you can use another sea vegetable, such as dulse flakes.

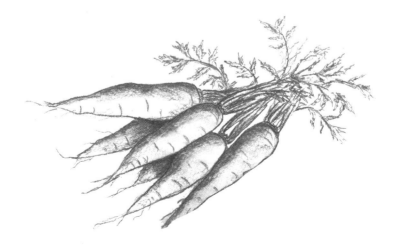

## VEGETABLES

# STEAMED GREENS
Serves 3 to 4

*Green leafy vegetables are loaded with calcium and other minerals and vitamins. Enjoy them at every meal. Serve them hot as a side dish or as a room-temperature salad with the Tofu Dressing found on page 88.*

| |
|---|
| 1 bunch of kale or other green leafy vegetable |
| $^1/_2$ cup spring water |
| Pinch of sea salt |

**Preparation:** Wash the kale and slice into $1^1/_2$-inch-long pieces, or cook them whole and cut after they are done. Add 1 inch of water and a pinch of sea salt in a medium-sized pot, before placing the steamer. Add the greens, cover the pot, and boil for 3 to 5 minutes or until greens are tender.

**Variation:** Choose a different green daily, like collard, mustard greens, turnip greens, bok choy, watercress, dandelion leaves, turnip leaves, or Chinese cabbage. For added taste, sauté your greens in a small amount of light sesame or olive oil.

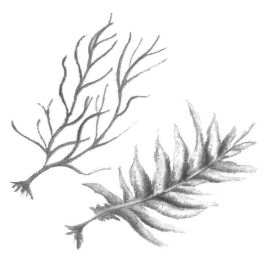

# ARAME SEA VEGETABLE DISH

Serves 4 to 5

*Arame sea vegetable is rich in minerals and traditionally used to help relieve female disorders. It's a perfect side dish for any meal and can be eaten up to three times per week.*

| |
|---|
| 1 cup arame sea vegetable |
| $1/2$ cup onions |
| 1 cup carrots |
| Cold spring water, to cover the vegetables |
| 2 tablespoons soy sauce or wheat-free tamari |
| 1 tablespoon umeboshi plum vinegar or lemon juice |
| 1 teaspoon light sesame oil or extra virgin olive oil |
| Scallions, sliced for garnish |

**Preparation:** Wash and drain the arame. Dice the onions and slice the carrots finely. Then, heat the oil in a skillet. Add the onions and sauté them for 2 minutes. Place the arame on top of the onions and add the carrots. Do not mix. Add spring water to half cover the arame sea vegetable and about $1/2$ tablespoon of soy sauce. Cover and simmer for about 15 minutes. Season to taste with soy sauce and umeboshi plum vinegar or lemon juice. Mix and simmer until liquid has evaporated. Place in a serving bowl and garnish.

**Variation:** Use hiziki sea vegetable instead of arame and cook slightly longer. Choose different root vegetables to add balance to your meal plan. Substitute sea salt and black pepper for the soy sauce.

# SWEET CABBAGE, SQUASH, and ONIONS

Serves 3 to 4

*These sweet-tasting vegetables are a delight. They will also strengthen your spleen, which is involved in the body's immune responses.*

| |
|---|
| $1/2$ cup cabbage |
| $1/2$ cup squash |
| $1/4$ cup onions |
| $1/4$-inch strip of kombu |
| 2 tablespoons of soy sauce or tamari, or $1/4$ teaspoon sea salt |
| 1 cup spring water |

**Preparation:** First cut the cabbage, squash, and onions into large chunks. Then take the kombu strip and soak it before cutting it into small strips. Place these strips in the bottom of a heavy pan. Layer onions, cabbage, and squash on top of the kombu. Add spring water to cover half of the vegetables and add soy sauce. Cover and bring to a boil, then lower the flame and simmer for 15 to 20 minutes, or until all the water is absorbed and the vegetables are soft. Serve hot.

**Variation:** Add any kind of root vegetables, shiitake mushrooms, or green cabbage to this dish.

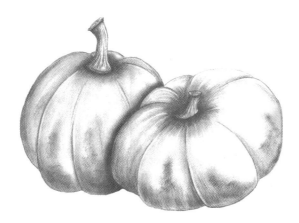

# LEAFY GREEN VEGETABLE ROLL

Serves 2

*Inspired by my love for Japanese nori rolls, this vegetable roll tastes so yummy that even children will eat it. You will need a sushi bamboo mat for this recipe.*

| |
|---|
| 1 bunch collard, whole leaves |
| 1 bunch napa (Chinese cabbage), whole leaves |
| 1 bag of sprouts, raw or slightly steamed |
| $^1/_4$ teaspoon of umeboshi plum paste |
| Sesame seeds, toasted as garnish |

**Preparation:** Boil whole leaves of vegetables in water for a few minutes. Cool them and place 3 leaves of collard on a sushi bamboo mat. Place 3 Chinese cabbage leaves on top of the collard leaves. Then spread the umeboshi paste evenly in a line, and add a few sprouts. Roll the vegetables into a cylinder and press out the liquid. Cut the roll into even pieces. Arrange them on a serving platter, add a few sprinkles of sesame seeds, and serve.

**Variation:** You can roll basically anything within these vegetables. Try carrots, scallions, pan-fried tofu, or even cooked beans or grains. Enjoy and be creative. Not that you need more heat in your food while going through menopause, but a horseradish dip will clean your head.

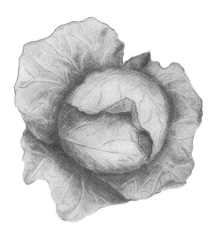

## SALADS

# WAKAME and CUCUMBER SALAD

Serves 3 to 4

*Raw cucumber is very cooling and can bring relief during hot flashes. Wakame is high in iron, calcium, vitamins A and C, niacin, and protein. Small amounts can be eaten daily in soups or salads. It is a Japanese delicacy.*

| |
|---|
| 2 cups cucumber |
| 2 tablespoons wakame |
| 1 tablespoon soy sauce, or $^1/_3$ tsp of sea salt |
| 2 tablespoons umeboshi plum vinegar or lemon juice |
| 1–2 sprigs of scallions |

**Preparation:** Slice the cucumbers; dice the white and green parts of the scallions; and soak and then slice the wakame. Combine cucumber, wakame, and scallions in a mixing bowl. Add soy sauce and umeboshi plum vinegar or lemon. Marinate for about $^1/_2$ hour before serving.

**Variation:** Press the salad with a heavy weight for $^1/_2$ hour, and use dulse flakes instead of wakame.

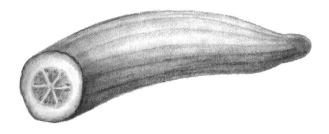

# SWEET and SOUR CARROT SALAD

Serves 3 to 4

*Sweet and Sour Carrot Salad is another very delicious raw salad, and one of my favorite potluck dishes. Carrots and apples provide soothing energy when you are feeling hot.*

| |
|---|
| 4 carrots |
| 1 apple, green or red |
| $1/4$ cup currants |
| 1 lemon, juiced |
| 2 tablespoons of umeboshi plum vinegar or apple cider vinegar |
| 3 tablespoons soy sauce, or $1/3$ teaspoon sea salt |
| 2 teaspoons rice syrup |

**Preparation:** Soak the currants in cold water for 5 to 7 minutes. Grate the carrots and the apple. Mix them together and add the currants. Add lemon juice, umeboshi plum vinegar, soy sauce, and rice syrup, and stir. Let the salad marinate in a cool place for up to $1/2$ hour, and serve.

**Variation:** Use $1/2$ cup of daikon radish instead of an apple for this dish. Replace the currants with raisins or other dried fruits.

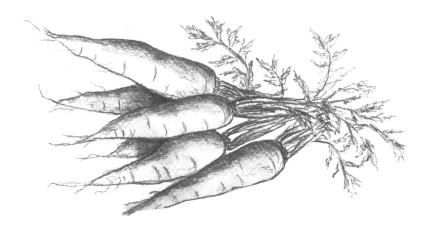

# BROCCOLI DELIGHT

Serves 3 to 4

*Broccoli, with its bright green color and flower-like texture, is a vegetable one can never overeat. Enjoy it often and serve it with your favorite meals. Eating broccoli supports the stomach, spleen, and lung energy.*

| |
|---|
| 3 cups of broccoli |
| 6 sprigs of scallions |
| 2 stalks celery |
| $3/4$ cup seedless grapes |
| $1/2$ cup almonds |
| **DRESSING** |
| $1/2$ cup rice milk |
| 2 tablespoons rice syrup |
| 1 tablespoon of umeboshi plum vinegar, rice vinegar, or apple cider vinegar |
| 1 tablespoon mustard |
| Pinch of sea salt |

**Preparation:** Slice the broccoli into small pieces; finely slice the celery and the white and green parts of the scallions; cut the grapes in half; and soak and lightly toast the almonds before cutting them into thin pieces. Steam the broccoli and celery for 2 minutes each and let them cool. Mix the slightly steamed broccoli and celery with the raw scallions, grapes, and toasted almonds. Combine the dressing ingredients and mix with a whisk or a fork and pour over the vegetables. Lightly toss and marinate for $1/2$ hour. Serve at room temperature.

**Variation:** The broccoli and celery can be eaten raw in this dish. You can use soy milk instead of rice milk, and lemon juice instead of umeboshi plum vinegar.

# GREENS with HIZIKI

Serves 4 to 5

*Rich in minerals, hiziki is a dark brown sea vegetable that turns black when dried. While soaking, it can expand to double or triple its size. It has a wiry consistency and is strong tasting. It grows native to Japan and the North Atlantic.*

| |
|---|
| 1/4 cup hiziki sea vegetable |
| 2 tablespoons soy sauce or tamari, or 1/4 teaspoons sea salt |
| 1 tablespoon umeboshi plum vinegar or lemon |
| 1 bunch collard greens |
| 2 carrots |
| 2 cups daikon |
| Scallions, finely cut, as garnish |
| **DRESSING** |
| 1 tablespoon extra virgin olive oil |
| 2 tablespoons rice vinegar or lemon |
| 2 tablespoons white or mellow miso, diluted with a little warm spring water |

**Preparation:** Wash, soak 20 minutes, and drain the hiziki. Wash and finely cut the collard greens. Wash and cut the carrots and the daikon julienne style. Boil hiziki in water with soy sauce-and-umeboshi plum vinegar mixture for 20 to 40 minutes. Remove and let cool. Steam the greens, carrots, and daikon separately. Let the vegetables cool down to room temperature, or rinse them under cold water. Combine hiziki and vegetables and add the rice vinegar, miso liquid, and olive oil. Mix well and let marinate for 1/2 hour. Serve at room temperature and garnish with scallions.

**Variation:** Choose different greens like kale, mustard greens, or broccoli, or use arame sea vegetable instead of hiziki. Add garlic or ginger to modify the strong taste of hiziki.

## DRESSINGS

# TOFU DRESSING

Serves 4 to 6

*A delicious dressing that can be used on salads, boiled vegetables, noodles, or sea vegetable dishes. Store it in a cool place for up to five days.*

| |
|---|
| 1 pound soft tofu |
| $\frac{1}{2}$ tablespoon of brown rice vinegar |
| 4 tablespoons of soy sauce, or to taste |
| 1 teaspoon of extra virgin olive oil |
| 1 cup spring water |

**Preparation:** Cut the tofu into large pieces. Boil it in spring water with the soy sauce for 5 minutes. Drain the excess liquid from the tofu. Blend the tofu with all the other ingredients in a blender or food processor until smooth.

**Variation:** Simmer the tofu in a miso paste for 5 minutes. Add ginger juice, herbs such as basil or chives, or a small piece of avocado for a change of flavors and color.

# TAHINI MISO DRESSING

Serves 2 to 3

*Tahini is a thick, smooth paste made from ground sesame seeds. Serve this dressing over cooked or raw vegetables, or as a dip or spread.*

| |
|---|
| 2 tablespoons of light miso |
| 1 tablespoon tahini |
| $1/2$ teaspoon tamari, soy sauce, or a pinch of sea salt |
| $1/2$ teaspoon lemon juice |
| Spring water, as needed |

**Preparation:** Add the light miso, tahini, tamari, lemon juice, and water into a suribachi or food processor. Blend all ingredients until smooth and creamy.

**Variation:** You can add chopped basil, parsley, or chives to the mixture. Use barley, chickpeas, or rice miso instead of a light miso.

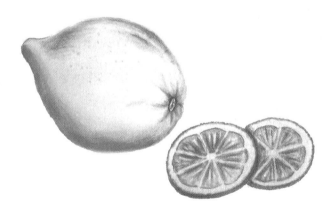

# SESAME DRESSING

Serves 4 to 5

*Sesame seeds are rich in protein, calcium, iron, and B vitamins. Sesame tea is good to darken the hair and treat menstrual irregularity. Sesame-ginger oil is good for arthritis, rheumatism, and ear ailments. This dressing will enhance a raw salad or cooked green leafy vegetable with its nutty taste of sesame seeds.*

| |
|---|
| 2 teaspoons light sesame oil |
| $1/2$ cup celery |
| $1/2$ cup scallions, white part |
| 1 tablespoon tamari or soy sauce or $1/3$ teaspoon of rock salt |
| 1 tablespoon of umeboshi plum vinegar, or lemon, rice, or apple cider vinegar |
| 2 tablespoons sesame seeds |
| $1/4$ teaspoon sea salt |
| 2 cups spring water |

**Preparation:** Finely dice both the celery and the white part of the scallions. Wash the sesame seeds and let them drip-dry in a strainer. In a skillet, toast the sesame seeds until slightly browned. Then grind in a suribachi. Lightly sauté the onions and celery in sesame oil until translucent. Add the salt, tamari, and umeboshi vinegar, and stir. Then slowly add the 2 cups of water and toasted sesame seeds, and bring everything to a quick boil. Remove from the stove and mix with vegetables. This dressing can be stored in a cool place and used on a raw salad or over cooked greens.

**Variation:** Sauté the vegetables with water and use 2 teaspoons of water instead of oil. Use a dash of raw dark sesame oil at the end to enhance the flavor.

# CREAMY LEMON GINGER DRESSING

Serves 4

*Use this dressing over a grain dish or over cooked and raw vegetable dishes.*

| |
|---|
| 2 teaspoons ginger juice |
| 3 tablespoons fresh lemon juice |
| 3 tablespoons extra virgin olive oil |
| 3 tablespoons flaxseed oil |
| 2 tablespoons spring water |
| 2 tablespoons scallions, white part |
| 1 teaspoon sea salt or Himalayan salt |
| 4 ounces soft tofu |
| Water-and-soy sauce mixture |

**Preparation:** Finely chop the white part of the scallions. Cut soft tofu into cubes and boil it in a water-and-soy sauce mixture for about 4 minutes. Place all the ingredients in a food processor and blend until smooth and creamy.

**Variation:** Choose from a variety of fresh or dried garden herbs like parsley, chives, rosemary, sage, or thyme to change the flavor of the dressing. Try using different oils.

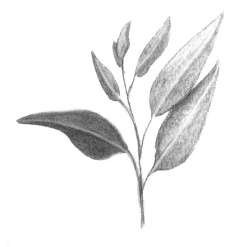

# GREEN LIFE DRESSING

Serves 4 to 5

*Use as a dip for vegetables. Avocados contain oleic acid, a monounsaturated fat that may help lower cholesterol. Avocados are a good source of potassium, a mineral that helps regulate blood pressure.*

| |
|---|
| 2 avocados |
| 4 ounces soft tofu |
| 7 sprigs of basil |
| 1 lemon, juice and rind |
| $1/4$ teaspoon sea salt |
| Spring water, small amount; optional |
| Extra virgin olive oil, small amount; optional |
| Water-and-soy sauce mixture |

**Preparation:** Cube the soft tofu. Then boil it in the water-and-soy sauce mixture. Clean and finely cut the sprigs of basil. Peel avocados and remove the seeds. Use soft green flesh and mix all ingredients in a blender or food processor. Purée until smooth while adding optional water or oil. Serve at room temperature.

**Variation:** Include a variety of finely chopped raw or steamed vegetables for different color and taste.

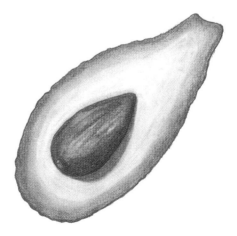

# PRESSED SALAD

Serves 5 to 7

*Eat a Pressed Salad as a side dish three to four times a week with a complete meal.*

| |
|---|
| 8 cups romaine hearts |
| 2 cups chicory salad |
| 2 tablespoons umeboshi plum vinegar or apple cider vinegar |
| $1/2$ teaspoon rice vinegar |
| 1 tablespoon soy sauce; optional |
| 1 tablespoon dulse flakes |
| $1/2$ teaspoon sea salt |

**Preparation:** Wash the romaine hearts and the chicory salad and cut into $1/2$-inch pieces. Then mix all ingredients together. Press with a plate and a heavy weight, or in a salad press, for about $1/2$ hour. There is no harm in letting the salad press longer if needed.

**Variation:** Try using different kinds of green leafy salads or vegetables to make a pressed salad. Add carrots, chives, or scallions. Use lemon juice instead of vinegar.

*Fermented Dishes*

# PICKLED RADISHES

Serves 5 to 7

*Serve often as a side dish with grain, beans, and cooked vegetables.*

| |
| --- |
| 2 cups radishes |
| 3 stems of scallions |
| 2 tablespoons dulse |
| 5 tablespoons carrots |
| 4 tablespoons rice vinegar, to taste |
| $^1/_3$ tsp sea salt |

**Preparation:** Slice the radishes and scallions; cut the carrots into matchstick-shaped pieces. Wash and soak the dulse, and then cut. Combine vegetables and place in a salad press. Add sea salt and vinegar to taste and mix. Press and let sit for a couple of hours before serving. These pickles keep for about one week if kept in a cool place.

**Variation:** Use white daikon radish or turnips. Add sea vegetables like dulse or nori flakes to the mixture. Use lemon juice, umeboshi plum vinegar, or apple cider vinegar instead of rice vinegar.

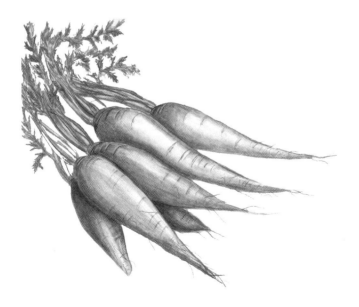

# HOMEMADE SAUERKRAUT

Serves 7 to 8

*Cabbage, a member of the crucifer family, is related to kale, broccoli, collards, and Brussels sprouts, and has similar benefits. Sauerkraut is a fermented cabbage dish, and can be eaten on a regular basis to strengthen the digestive system.*

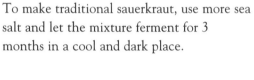

2 cups white cabbage

1 teaspoon sea salt, or less

**Preparation:** Shred the white cabbage. Mix and slightly press the cabbage with sea salt in a deep bowl. Place a plate with a heavy weight on top of the cabbage. Let sit and ferment for at least a couple of hours before serving. This dish stays fresh in a cool place for about one week.

**Variation:** Use a salad press for quick pickling. Add shredded carrots or daikon, chives, parsley, or scallions to the mixture for variation. Use umeboshi plum vinegar, rice vinegar, or apple cider vinegar and adjust the amount of sea salt.

To make traditional sauerkraut, use more sea salt and let the mixture ferment for 3 months in a cool and dark place.

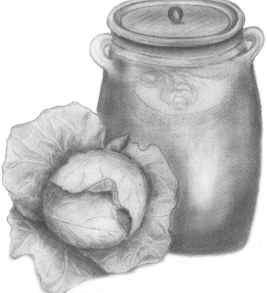

## FISH

# VEGETABLE STIR FRY with FISH

Serves 3 to 5

*Serve as a side dish with Brown Rice (page 67) and a Wakame and Cucumber Salad (page 84).*

| |
|---|
| 1–2 tablespoons extra virgin olive oil |
| $^1/_2$ onion |
| 2 cloves of garlic |
| 1 pound of fresh and firm white meat fish |
| Pinch of sea salt and black pepper |
| 1 cup carrots |
| 1 cup cauliflower |
| 1 cup broccoli, stems and heads |
| 2–3 tablespoons soy sauce, or to taste; optional |
| 1 cup spring water or vegetable broth |
| Scallion, sliced for garnish |

**Preparation:** Cut the onion into thin slices; mince the garlic; wash, dry, and cut the white meat fish into cubes; cut the cauliflower into very small florets; cut the carrots julienne style; and cut the broccoli into small pieces. Heat oil gently in a stainless steel wok or large pan. Quickly sauté onion for 1 minute, then add garlic, stirring for a few seconds. Move the garlic and onions to the side, and add fish and season with sea salt. Gently sauté the fish until browned on all sides, then stir together with garlic and onions, and season with a few drops of soy sauce. Remove from pot and set aside. Quickly sauté carrots and cauliflower, adding more oil, and season with salt and pepper. Add a small amount of water, cover, and simmer for 4 minutes. Then add the broccoli and fish you set aside, mix, and simmer for 2 minutes. Add small amounts of water to prevent burning. Mix all ingredients gently and add more seasoning, if needed. Garnish with sliced scallions and serve hot. Serve grated daikon with a drop of soy sauce or a dash of lemon on the side.

**Variation:** Choose different vegetables, like snow peas, celery, and water chestnuts, or add shiitake, chanterelle, or maitake mushrooms. Add ginger juice, to taste. Prepare a vegetarian stir fry using tofu or other cooked beans like chickpeas instead of fish. Add kudzu to thicken the sauce. Use shrimp, Northern pink or spot prawns from Newfoundland, or organically farm-raised tilapia.

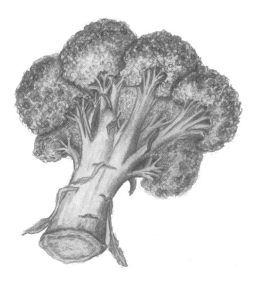

# SALMON with PESTO

Serves 1

*Serve the salmon, an omega-3-fatty-acid-rich fish, with freshly steamed green leafy vegetables and a light grain or noodle dish. I thank my friend and chef Michelle Licata for this wonderful recipe.*

| |
|---|
| 4–6 ounce salmon per person, wild caught from Alaska |
| 2 tablespoons of pesto (a basil, olive oil, and pine nut blend) |
| Sprig of parsley, for garnish |

**Preparation:** Place salmon skin down in an oiled pan and spread the pesto evenly over the salmon. Roast the salmon in a preheated 400°F oven for 15 to 20 minutes. Or, use an instant-read thermometer and remove the salmon when it has reached 120°F. Serve hot and garnish with a sprig of parsley. Serve grated daikon with a drop of soy sauce on the side.

**Variation:** Marinate the salmon—or a white meat fish—in a water-and-soy sauce mixture for one hour and bake or quick-broil. Add garlic, ginger juice, or garden herbs like rosemary to the mixture. Prepare an umeboshi plum sauce with kudzu to serve with the fish.

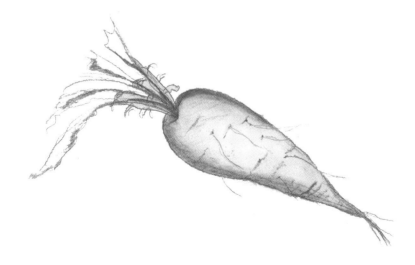

# POACHED FISH in WHITE WINE

Serves 1

*Serve this dish with boiled brown basmati rice, steamed carrots, and a bed of fresh salad greens.*

| |
|---|
| 4–6-ounce halibut per person, wild caught from Alaska |
| $^1/_2$ cup white wine |
| $^1/_3$ cup water |
| $^1/_3$ teaspcon of sea salt |
| Sprig of rosemary, for garnish |

**Preparation:** Wash and dry fish. Heat the pan and place the fish skin side down. Add wine, some water, and salt. Bring the mixture quickly to a boil, then reduce heat and simmer for 10 to 15 minutes while partially uncovered. The alcohol from the wine will evaporate, but the taste will remain. Serve with a sprig of rosemary for garnish, and drizzle some of the remaining liquid over the fish. Serve grated daikon with a drop of soy sauce on the side.

**Variation:** Thicken the remaining liquid with kudzu. Add garlic, rosemary, scallions, or chives as seasonings. Prepare this dish by sautéing the fish before adding the liquid. Use Mirin (a sweet Japanese wine), red wine, or just spring water, instead of the white wine. For a sweet caramelized taste add one teaspoon of maple syrup to the liquid and simmer. Marinate the fish in a water-and-soy sauce mixture for $^1/_2$ hour before poaching.

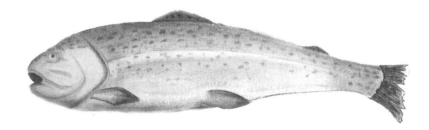

# SUSHI MAKI ROLL

Makes 1 roll

*Sushi Maki Rolls are great party finger foods. Involve your guests and let them roll their own. Serve them for lunch or as an anytime snack for your family. You will need a sushi bamboo mat for this recipe.*

| |
|---|
| 1 sheet of sushi nori, toasted |
| 1 cup of rice, white or brown <br> (see Brown Rice recipe on page 67) |
| 1 tablespoon of sushi vinegar (heated mixture of rice <br> vinegar, water, and rice syrup, to taste) |
| **SUSHI FILLING PER ROLL** |
| 2–3 slices of sushi-grade salmon or tuna, wild caught <br> from Alaska |
| Dash of wasabi powder (a Japanese horseradish) |
| 1 strip of carrot, slightly steamed |
| 1 strip of scallion, slightly steamed |

**Preparation:** Cook brown or white rice as instructed in Brown Rice recipe. Put cooked rice in a bowl and pour sushi vinegar evenly over the surface, mixing into rice with quick cutting strokes. Put a sheet of nori, shiny side down, on a sushi bamboo mat. Place the prepared sushi rice on the nori sheet and press down, leaving $1/4$ inch free on top and bottom. Do not pack rice; rolling will take care of that. Rice should be less than $1/4$ inch thick. Be careful not to use too much rice. Dilute a dash of wasabi power with cold water to form a paste. Put this paste in one horizontal line in the middle of the rice. Place a carrot strip, scallion, and slices of fish in one line, on top. Slowly fold the mat over, tucking the end of nori to start a roll. Keep lifting up the mat as you go. Lessen pressure slightly to straighten out the roll, if needed. Continue rolling with medium pressure. Roll up and wet the empty place on the nori, to hold it together. Remove sushi roll from mat and cut into 6 or 8 even pieces with a wet knife. Serve with a soy sauce-wasabi dip, grated white daikon radish with a drop of soy sauce, and ginger pickles on the side.

**Variation:** Roll a vegetarian Sushi Maki and use a variety of vegetables, fried tofu, tempeh, or seitan (a wheat product that tastes like meat) instead of fish. Apply umeboshi plum paste instead of wasabi paste on the rice. Add smoked salmon instead of raw, or use a variety of sushi-grade fish to make a Sushi Maki Roll.

# DESSERTS

SWEET TOFU CREAM
COUSCOUS CAKE
RICE PUDDING
ORANGE CREAM with STRAWBERRIES

*Desserts*

# SWEET TOFU CREAM

Serves 2 to 3

*Yummy, yummy. As an occasional treat, tofu can be prepared with a sweetener.*

| |
|---|
| 1 pack of very soft tofu |
| $1/4$ cup soymilk or ricemilk, or less |
| 1 cup berries, fresh or frozen; your choice |
| 3 tablespoons rice syrup, barley malt, or maple syrup |
| Pinch of sea salt |
| Fresh mint and fruit, as garnish |

**Preparation:** Mix all the ingredients in a blender or food processor until smooth. Serve in a decorative bowl and garnish each serving with fresh fruit and a leaf of mint.

**Variation:** Instead of fresh or frozen berries use 3 teaspoons of grain coffee. Use a variety of locally grown fruits. Include almond butter, sesame tahini, or peanut butter in your blend and omit the berries. You can also boil the tofu first, then let it cool down, before you put it in the blender.

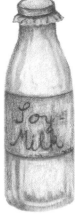

# COUSCOUS CAKE

Serves 4 to 5

*If you are allergic to wheat, you can substitute couscous with quinoa or millet. Watch for different cooking times of the grains.*

| |
|---|
| 1 cup whole grain couscous |
| 2 cups apple juice |
| 1 cup blueberries, or fruit of your choice |
| Pinch of sea salt |
| $1/2$ cup walnuts, slightly toasted for garnish |

**Preparation:** Bring apple juice to a boil and add salt. Turn heat off and first add the blueberries, then the couscous. Stir gently and cover with a lid. After about 10 minutes, or when the liquid has been absorbed, place the couscous mixture in a glass mold. Let cool and invert it on a serving dish. Serve with Sweet Tofu Cream (page 101) and toasted walnuts.

**Variation:** Add a kudzu juice glaze on top of the cooled cake. Dissolve 2 tablespoons of kudzu in 1 cup of cold juice of your choice. Add a pinch of sea salt and bring the mixture slowly to a boil. Stir constantly until it thickens, and pour it over the cake. Either serve while the kudzu juice is still warm and creamy, or wait until it is cool and hardened.

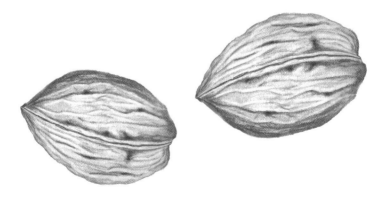

# RICE PUDDING

Serves 4 to 5

*Want a nourishing dessert? You have to try this one.*

| |
|---|
| 2 cups organic brown rice, already cooked (see Brown Rice recipe on page 67) |
| $^1/_2$ cup raisins, soaked and chopped |
| $^1/_2$ cup almonds, toasted and slivered |
| 2 cups apple juice, or more if needed |
| 4 cloves |
| 2 cinnamon sticks |
| 1 teaspoon kudzu, dissolved in 2 teaspoons cold spring water |
| $^1/_4$ cup almonds |

**Preparation:** Heat apple juice with cloves and cinnamon sticks. Remove after juice has come to a boil. Add the cooked brown rice and raisins to the juice and simmer for about 20 minutes. Toast the almonds in the oven at 250°F until slightly brown and add to the pudding. Pour dissolved kudzu into the pudding and stir until it thickens. Serve hot and garnish with a few toasted almonds.

**Variation:** Place the pudding in a baking pan and bake at 250°F in a pre-heated stove for about 20 minutes. Remove, let cool, and invert. Then serve as a cake.

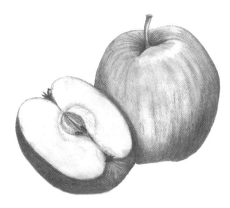

# ORANGE CREAM
# with STRAWBERRIES

Serves 4 to 5

*This is a very soothing and satisfying dessert, and is quick to make.*

| |
| --- |
| 1 pint of strawberries |
| 2 cups orange juice |
| 2 teaspoons rice syrup |
| 4 drops vanilla |
| Pinch of sea salt |
| 3 teaspoons of kudzu, dissolved in a little cold water |
| Pinch of cinnamon, as garnish |
| Mint leaves, as garnish |

**Preparation:** Clean the strawberries and cut into fourths. Bring 2 cups of orange juice with a pinch of sea salt to a boil. Add the rice syrup and vanilla, and simmer for a minute. Add dissolved kudzu while stirring constantly for 3 minutes, until the kudzu thickens. At this point add the cut and cleaned strawberries, and let simmer on a low flame for 1 to 2 minutes. Serve hot and decorate with a touch of cinnamon and leaves of fresh mint.

**Variation:** Instead of orange juice, prepare this dessert with apple juice or any other unsweetened juice. Choose different berries or tree fruits, like apples or pears. Boil the juice with a cinnamon stick and remove it before serving. Decorate with lemon or orange zest.

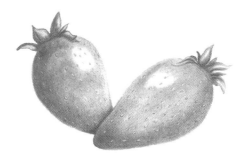

# THE NATURAL PANTRY

All items in your pantry should be organically grown. Shop at natural food stores—such as Whole Foods Market—or order your groceries from Eden Foods, Goldmine, or the Kushi Store. For more information on these stores and other providers of traditionally made, quality macrobiotic products, see the Resources section on page 129.

## BEANS

Adzuki Beans

Black Soybeans

Chickpeas – Garbanzo

Lentils – Green and Brown

## BEAN PRODUCTS

Natto

Tempeh

Tofu – Fresh and Dry

## BEVERAGES

Bancha – Roasted Leaf Tea

Barley – Grain Coffee

Green Tea

Green Tea with Brown Rice

Kukicha – Roasted Stem Tea

## CONDIMENTS

Gomasio

Nori Flakes

Shiso Leaf Powder

Tekka

## COOKWARE

Stainless Steel, Glass, Ceramic, or Cast Iron

Ceramic Grater

Mac Vegetable Knife

Pickle Press

Pressure Cooker

Suribachi and Pestle

Sushi Bamboo Mat

Wooden Cutting Board and Utensils

## WHOLE GRAINS

Barley

Brown Rice – Short, Medium, Long

Corn

Hato Mugi – Wild Barley

Kamut

Millet

Quinoa

Rice – Sweet and Wild

Whole Oats

## PICKLES

Ginger Pickles

Raw Sauerkraut

Takuan – Daikon Radish Pickle

## SEASONINGS

Kudzu

Mirin

Miso, Barley, Rice – Aged Two Years

Miso – Light or Mellow, Rice, Barley,
   Chickpeas – Aged 3 months

Cold Pressed Extra Virgin Olive Oil

Black Pepper

Himalayan Crystal Salt

Sea Salt – White, Unbleached

Sesame Oil – Dark and Light

Soy Sauce – Alcohol Free

Wheat-Free Tamari

Umeboshi Plum, Paste and Vinegar

Rice Vinegar, Apple Cider Vinegar

## SEA VEGETABLES

Arame

Dulse Flakes

Hiziki

Kombu

Nori

Nori Flakes

Wakame

## SEEDS AND NUTS

Almonds

Flax Seeds

Pumpkin Seeds

Sesame Seeds

Sunflower Seeds

Walnuts

## SWEETENERS

Amazake

Apple Juice

Barley Malt

Brown Rice Syrup

Maple Syrup

# STORIES and PORTRAITS

Marquita Wepman

Monica Feifel

Rosangélica Aburto

Shizuko Yamamoto

Sylvia Lemus Sharma

Susun S. Weed

# MARQUITA WEPMAN

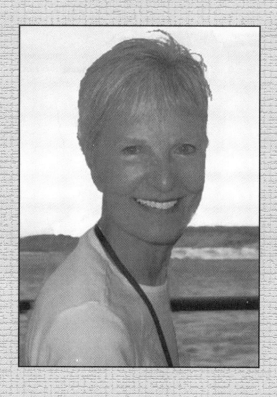

*I* have three children and six grandchildren.

My menses began just before my thirteenth birthday. It came every twenty-eight days, and would last for a week. I flowed for five days and then had two light days for the process to close down.

At the age of forty-five, I began practicing macrobiotics. The first year, my menses continued as one long period for five months. During the next four years, I occasionally ate dairy products, desserts, and caffeinated drinks. When I became serious about macrobiotics and stopped eating dairy food, fasted, and did yoga and acupuncture, the fibroid tumors which I had had for thirty years detached from my uterus and were discharged.

From my late forties to fifty-seven, I went through menopause. At the beginning, I began to experience irregular periods, with heavy flowing. At times I felt depressed, unsure of myself and upset. Feelings I had not felt since my years in therapy.

Most of my woman friends were younger than I, and without a woman in my family who had gone through menopause naturally, I had no one to talk to. My mother, aunts, and sister had all had hysterectomies. After reading a handful of books on menopause, I was appalled to learn that a huge percentage of hysterectomies are totally unnecessary.

When I asked my teacher, Aveline Kushi, about her menopause, she compared her experience to a hurricane—a tremendous upheaval during the process, followed by a beautiful and peaceful serenity afterward. I have learned that diet and lifestyle, choices over which I have a marked degree of control, influence my experience of life.

The macrobiotic teachings of the Five Energy Transformation Theory, which can also be applied to a woman's life cycle, helped me to understand this. The floating water energy of winter represents a woman's gestation as an embryo inside the womb; the upward energy of spring represents the young female being born out into the world; the active energy of summer represents the ripening of maidenhood and her menarche; the downward energy of late summer represents the maturation of a woman's reproductive organs, maintaining nourishment for her fertile ovarian cycle and the opportunity of motherhood; and the gathering and contracting energy of fall represents the shrinking of her ovaries, thereby depleting her supply of follicles and eggs (ovum), and closing down, drying up, of her menstrual cycle. Thus menopause.[1] [© Marquita Wepman]

Having gone through menopause naturally, without any artificial assistance, has given me physical, as well as spiritual and emotional, strengths. My feeling of freedom to pursue new ideas without fear of "being too old" is fueled by such strength. I feel mature and experienced, young and adventurous, at different times.

MONICA FEIFEL

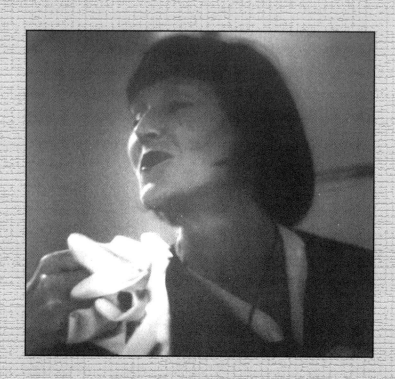

*I* was born in Germany, lived fifteen years in the US, and moved back to Germany during my menopausal passage. I have a sixteen-year-old daughter.

My first symptoms of menopause were hourly hot flashes that woke me in the night. These I had for years before my periods stopped at age forty-four. There were other symptoms, like mood changes, concentration problems, memory problems, dryness of mucous membranes, and decreased libido. My doctor said that stress and smoking could bring on menopause early. It was quite a shock, because I wasn't well informed.

The frequent hot flashes caused a nervous condition, which affected my work. The doctors advised me to take hormones—the estrogen from horse urine, and progestin. In two weeks, the hot flashes stopped completely, and I was feeling much better. The months following, I developed water retention and abnormal appetite. I ate like a horse. So, I stopped the hormones. After awhile, the hot flashes and all the other symptoms came back.

I checked into alternative health care and tried different teas and herbs for several months, but none of them helped me. The synthetic estrogen I tried seemed to have no side effects, but then, after awhile, it did. For more than two years, I went back and forth with hormones, or no hormones, and teas, homeopathic products, progesterone creams, and herbs. I got no relief. In fact, the hot flashes became worse.

When I moved to Germany I saw by chance a woman's herbal tea in a health food store. After two weeks of drinking at least two cups of tea per day, the hot flashes stopped. Sometimes I still have really light ones. I'm not sure if it was the tea, but in any case, I want to share the herbal tea mixture, which seemed to help me.

## MENOPAUSAL HERBAL TEA MIXTURE FROM GERMANY

| $1\frac{1}{2}$ teaspoons Walnut Leaves |
| --- |
| 2 tablespoons Rosemary |
| $1\frac{1}{2}$ teaspoons Avens |
| $\frac{1}{2}$ teaspoon Lady's Mantle |
| 5 teaspoons St. Joan's Wort |
| 7 teaspoons Yarrow |
| 1 teaspoon White Archangel |

**Preparation:** Bring spring water to a boil and turn off the heat. To 1 cup of water add 1 to 2 teaspoons of the tea mixture. Cover and let steep for about 10 to 15 minutes. Strain and drink 1 cup three to four times a day.

Problems with concentration when I read and memory loss at work continue to trouble me. If this mental change were common knowledge for men and women, and was accepted as a natural part of being human, perhaps it would be less painful.

# ROSANGÉLICA ABURTO

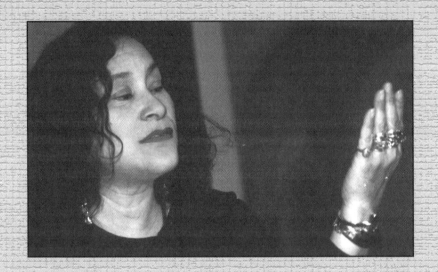

*I* was born in Nicaragua and moved to the United States when I was twenty-one years old. I am the oldest in my family, but I have no children of my own.

At that time my mother hadn't gone through menopause, so it was not an issue present in my family. But the women of menopausal age talked among themselves about it. I do remember men making jokes when a woman got upset. They would tease, saying, "Oh my goodness, she has hysteria, she must be going through the change." On a subconscious level, there was the idea that women were somehow less after menopause, because they couldn't bear children. This is a general sense of how menopause was dealt with in Nicaragua.

When I started menopause, I missed periods for two months. This was very unusual because all my life I had been like a clock. As I was celebrating my new freedom, I was surprised by another period. This time, I continued bleeding for three weeks.

The doctor told me that I was lacking estrogen and that I was menopausal. With 10 milligrams of just estrogen, the bleeding stopped, but only temporarily. This time my doctor recommended a hysterectomy as an alternative, which I felt was completely out of the question. As a drastic measure, a double dosage of birth control pills twice daily was prescribed to regulate my system. Reluctantly, I continued this treatment for three months, thinking my body would find its own regular rhythm. When I stopped taking birth control pills, the bleeding returned. My hemoglobin level dropped from 13 to the dangerous point of 9.8. I felt very ill.

My social life and work began to suffer. Looking at my history and genetic makeup, I found that I was not a high-risk candidate for breast cancer. My doctor insisted that Hormone Replacement Therapy was the most effective way to deal with my problem and alleviate the symptoms. As my body wouldn't regulate itself, I finally agreed. I began a combination of 5 milligrams provera for twelve days and 75 milligrams premarin daily. I still got my periods, but they were hormone induced and not as intense as during my reproductive years. Although I was reluctant to use artificial hormones at first, they have helped me with my menopausal symptoms of hemorrhaging. I continued using hormones for about five years, but stopped when I developed side effects.

My advice to women is to learn about possible menopausal symptoms and begin preventive measures early. If symptoms arise, stay active and eat healthy. Avoid a hysterectomy—they are often performed unnecessarily, and other ways to deal with symptoms are available. Talk to friends, support groups, and doctors, and make wise and rational decisions. Menopause is nothing to be ashamed of and nothing to hide from.

# SHIZUKO YAMAMOTO

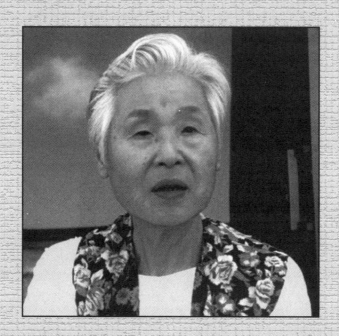

$\mathcal{I}$ was born in Japan and moved to the United States in the early sixties. I have no children.

My menstruation came naturally, with no complications. Menopause should have been the same. But of course, my body had changed with age. Before I began eating a macrobiotic diet, I had overloaded my spleen and pancreas with sugary, greasy, and cold foods.

I was forty-nine years old when I began my change of life. I noticed more psychological tension than physical problems. Hot and cold flashes at night lasted for two years. I took my blanket on and off all night long. These flashes went away little by little. When psychological difficulties emerged, I could not control my emotions and as a result I became anguished.

According to Oriental medicine, the spleen and pancreas are very important for overall health. They are located in the center of the body and are involved in the immune, hormonal, and psychological functions of the body. When these organs function well, mood swings and hot flashes should not be experienced during menopause. During my menopausal passage, these organs were not functioning well.

I have eaten a macrobiotic diet for over forty years. Physically, I am able to keep up, and at the same time, my mind is very peaceful. I am more peaceful now and not as anguished as when I went through menopause. This means that my spleen and pancreas energy is better now, at age seventy-two, than at age forty-nine. The healing of these organs occurred slowly over a period of time.

People often think, "If I change my diet, I will immediately get better." But they misunderstand. Macrobiotics is not like western medicine. A macrobiotic diet follows the rhythm of the seasons. A natural healing process occurs in harmony with nature's movement. We are part of nature; we are together.

Sometimes I wondered why I was eating a macrobiotic diet. Why was I trying so hard to cut out sugar, dairy, meat, and refined products? Now that I am older, I understand it better.

I have had many experiences with hospitals and operations. I don't want to go through them again at the end of my life. I do not want to die in a hospital. I want to die naturally, without pain or medicine, in my bed. When I was young I never thought about this. With more than two-thirds of my life over, I am focusing on a peaceful and happy life, and preparing for a smooth passage to death.

SYLVIA LEMUS SHARMA

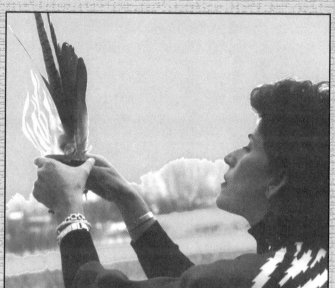

*I* am a Mexican living in Minnesota, United States. My husband and I have a son and a daughter.

My investigation into menopause began when my husband and I attended a menopause program sponsored by a pharmaceutical company. The female speaker described her experience as "coming down" with menopause. A young male gynecologist told the audience that he prescribed many women hormones, but they usually didn't continue taking them after three months.

A male doctor whom I consulted in regard to my fibroids recommended that I have a hysterectomy at the age of forty-three. He considered it a sensible option, as my reproductive years were over. Additionally, he thought it would alleviate the annoyance of my monthly blood clots. It did not feel right to have a hysterectomy for these reasons. In France, only the fibroids are removed, because it is considered important for women to keep their female organs. After hearing his advice, I found two female doctors who monitored my situation.

As I sought other healing practices, I became connected to women also seeking help with female issues. My search led me to the Native American Ojibwa traditional women. They invited me to a special women's lodge to experience their way of celebrating female strength and harmony for women in their moon. They explained that in their matriarchal society, women hold an honored place, as they are considered the first ones. We were all warrior women in harmony with the moon and the sun. We were fed first by everyone that weekend. It did not surprise me that I should get my moon on my visit to this place, and I experienced hot flashes for the first time in my life.

In the beginning of my menopausal journey I tried the conventional medical establishment. This was not what I needed. The ideology of the Ojibwa traditional women resonated with me and nurtured me through my passage. Through their stories I learned that I must go back to my own traditions. This I have done, by finding my heritage through the sacred dances of the ancient Aztec culture.

Many of my new friends are strong vibrant women who celebrate turning fifty. Some of us held a ceremony for my fiftieth birthday, at the pyramids in Chichen Itza in Mexico. After this celebration, I felt so strongly about honoring the circle of life through dance that I started a "Mexica" women's dance circle in the Midwest. I am grateful for the change in my life, and feel blessed to have found the connection to my tradition. I will continue my passage into old age and wisdom, dancing.

SUSUN S. WEED

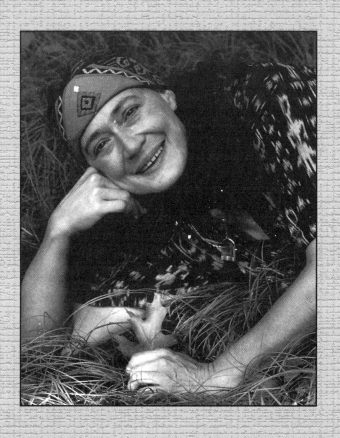

*In* 1990, at the age of forty-four, I began to think about menopause. Back then women didn't talk about menopause the way we do now. It was almost a taboo subject. When I asked my mother about her menopause she told me, "I threw away my unused pads." I knew there was more to it than that. I was curious; I was terrified.

I resolved to learn as much as I could about The Change, as soon as possible, and to write it all down. Somewhere I had heard that women "lost their minds" during menopause. By writing about it, at least I would have something to refer to that could help me when I lost my mind and memory during menopause.

I studied, read, dreamt, and wrote about menopause for two full years. I felt as though I was on a fast train hurtling toward an unknown destination, and I had to keep running or the train would fly out from under my feet. The more I read, the more I realized how little is known about menopause in healthy women.

When asking women to tell me about menopause and their experiences of it, I was shocked and thrilled. It was different from the scary rumors I'd heard and the grim pictures medical books had painted. While each woman had an individual story to tell, there was an overall theme: Menopause as the ultimate metamorphosis. Caterpillars, turned into butterflies. Post-menopausal women became powerful, truthful, potent, and vital.

No matter how hard I looked I couldn't find any missing hormones. Women are born making twenty-nine kinds of estrogen. These are baseline estrogens, which are basically the same every day of our lives. Between puberty and menopause, the thirtieth estrogen—estradiol—is produced, for one or two days a month, to trigger ovulation. Since estradiol is stronger than all the other estrogens combined, scientific medicine focuses on it. That's why they say that women stop making estrogen after menopause. Of course, women never stop making estrogen; we only stop making estradiol.

Estradiol acts to keep our life force (chi, kundalini) centered in our pelvis, uterus, and ovaries. When we stop making estradiol, chi is free to flow up the spine. When driven by powerful hot flashes, this creates an awakening, enlightenment if you will. No wonder they think menopausal women lose their minds. We do, in the best possible sense.

Menopause is a gateway to enlightenment. As the chi—in the form of hot flashes—moves up the spine, every gland in a woman's body shifts, changing her every aspect: physical, emotional, mental, sexual, and psychic. The healthier the woman, the more hot flashes she may have, and the more likely she will be able to use the energy of those flashes to build her health and wisdom.

Menopause is hard work, and tires most women out. But when it's over, if women have taken care of themselves during the Change, they find they have more power and energy than ever before.

Taking care of oneself is multidimensional, of course. It is nourishment in its broadest sense.

I urge women to take a Crone's Year Away during most of menopause meltdown, and drink nourishing herbal infusions. And to listen closely to their bodies regarding what foods they eat.

It came as no surprise to me to find the majority of vegetarian women eating meat during and after menopause. The Change is hard work. Animal protein is critically important to maintain bone and heart health and become an outrageous old woman. Soy—especially in the form of soy "milk," soy "cheese," soy "meats," soy "ice cream," and other contrived soy products— is one of the worst things a menopausal woman can do to herself.

Unfermented soy contains anti-nutritional substances, which bind calcium (weakening bones), zinc (interfering with immune strength), vitamin B12 (setting the stage for dementia), and thyroid hormone (depressing thyroid functioning). Miso and tamari don't, and their cancer-repelling abilities are well documented. I eat them daily.

Living in Manhattan in the mid-sixties as the proprietor of a "New Age" store I came into contact with macrobiotics. Though never a serious student, I was deeply attracted to the spiritual aspects of macrobiotics. From it I learned a reverence for rice, grain, and food. I saw that "eating what is in season" would assure me of the healthiest, least expensive, most ecologically sound food choices. The ultimate extension of that, to me, was to eat the wild foods that the earth provided.

The wild mushrooms (maitake, chanterelles) and wild meats (venison, turkey, and rabbit) supported my menopause and were gifted to me by the forest. My menopause was grounded by the wild roots (burdock, dandelion, yellow dock, chicory, Jerusalem artichoke) gifted to me from the byways. My menopause was powered by the wild weedy greens and flowers (nettle, red clover, linden, comfrey, lamb's quarter, amaranth) gifted to me by the meadows, by the peopled places. My menopause was eased by the wild medicines (motherwort, milk thistle, St. Joan's/John's Wort, skullcap, shepherd's purse, cleavers) gifted to me by the Green Nations.

In December of 1994, I had my last period. In between, I bled for thirty days. I was curious to see how long it would continue, and if it would stop on its own. But after a month, I was too tired to continue and took herbs, which stopped the bleeding within twenty-four hours. I could no longer tolerate a sip of wine without having massive flashes. Every baby I saw brought tears. Panting with heat, lying on the floor, I rode my hot flashes; slept in snatches, and observed, with awe, my body, mind, and soul's ability to transform. When it was all behind me, when I emerged from my cocoon, spread my butterfly wings, I received my Crone's Crowning.

Menopausal wisdom needs to be shared, woman-to-woman, for the health of each woman, and for the health of the planet. Dr. Kristen Hawkes, of the University of Utah, maintains that post-menopausal women have always been the ones who knew how to save both community and world when times were hard. With a little help from our friends, we can do it. Green blessings— from a wise woman and a green witch.

# GLOSSARY of TERMS

Excerpts are from *Aveline Kushi's Complete Guide to Macrobiotic Cooking.*

| | |
|---|---|
| **Adzuki Bean** | Small, dark red bean, grown originally in Japan but now also grown in the West. Also known as aduki bean. |
| **Amazake** | A sweet, creamy beverage made from fermented sweet brown rice. |
| **Arame** | A thin, wiry, black, and mineral-rich sea vegetable, similar to hiziki. |
| **Bancha Tea** | Twigs, stems, and leaves from mature Japanese tea bushes; also known as kukicha tea. |
| **Barley** | A whole cereal grain, and traditional staple of the Middle East and Southern Europe. |
| **Barley Malt** | A natural sweetener made from concentrated barley that has a rich, roasted taste. |
| **Bonito Flakes** | Flakes shaved from dried bonito fish. Used in soup stocks or as a garnish. |
| **Bran** | The outer coating of the whole grain together with the germ removed, during refining, to produce white flour or white rice. Bran may be used in pickling or as a garnish. |
| **Brown Rice** | Whole unpolished rice; comes in three main varieties: short, medium, and long grain. Brown rice contains an ideal balance of nutrients and is the principle staple in macrobiotic cooking. |
| **Cold Pressed** | Pertaining to oils processed at low temperatures to preserve their natural qualities. |

| | |
|---|---|
| Daikon | A long white radish used in many types of dishes and for medicinal purposes. |
| Dulse | A red-purple sea vegetable used in soups, salads, vegetable dishes, or as a garnish. |
| Gomasio | Sesame seed salt made from dry roasting and grinding sea salt and sesame seeds and crushing them in a Suribachi. |
| Hiziki | A dark brown sea vegetable which when dried turns black. It has a wiry consistency and may be strong tasting. Grows native to Japan and the North Atlantic. |
| Kombu | A wide, thick, dark sea vegetable that grows in deep ocean water. Used in making soup stocks, condiments, and candy, and cooked as a separate dish or with vegetables, beans, or grains. |
| Macrobiotics | From the traditional Greek word for Great Life or Long Life, this is the way of life according to the largest possible view, the infinite order of the universe. The practice of macrobiotics includes the understanding and practical application of the order of the universe in daily life. This includes the selection, preparation, and manner of cooking and eating, as well as the orientation of consciousness. |
| Millet | A small yellow grain that can be prepared whole, added to soups, salads, and vegetable dishes, or baked. It is a staple food of China and Africa. |
| Mirin | A sweet cooking wine made from sweet rice. |
| Miso | A fermented paste made from soybeans, sea salt, and usually rice or barley. Used in soups, stews, spreads, baking, and as seasoning, miso has a nice sweet taste and gives a salty flavor. |
| Natto | Cooked white soybeans and mixed with beneficial enzymes and fermented for twenty-four hours. This is a sticky dish, with long strands and a strong odor, and is good for improving digestion. |
| Natural Foods | Whole foods that are not processed or treated with artificial additives or preservatives. |
| Nori | Thin sheets of dried sea vegetable. Black or dark purple, they turn green when roasted over a flame. They can be used as a garnish, to wrap rice balls, in making sushi, or with tamari soy sauce as a condiment. |
| Organic Foods | Foods grown without the use of chemical fertilizers, herbicides, pesticides, genetic modified organism (GMO), or other artificial sprays. |

| | |
|---|---|
| Oxalic Acid | Found in plants; binds with calcium to form insoluble compounds, limiting the calcium that can be absorbed. |
| Pressed Salad | Salad prepared by pressing sliced vegetables and sea salt in a small pickle press or with an improvised weight. |
| Pressure Cooker | An airtight metal pot that cooks food quickly by steaming it under pressure at a high temperature. Used primarily in macrobiotic cooking for whole grains and occasionally for beans with vegetables. |
| Rice Syrup | A natural sweetener made from malted brown rice. |
| Sea Salt | Salt obtained from the ocean. Unlike refined table salt, unrefined sea salt is high in trace minerals and contains no chemicals, sugar, or added iodine. |
| Sea Vegetable | Edible vegetable from the seas such as kombu, wakame, arame, hiziki, nori, or dulse. Sea vegetables are rich in minerals. |
| Shiitake | A mushroom native to Japan but now cultivated in the United States as well. Used widely dried or fresh in cooking, for soups and stews, and in medical preparations. |
| Soba | Noodles made from buckwheat flour or buckwheat combined with whole wheat. |
| Soymilk | A liquid residue from cooking tofu. Used as beverage, often a milk substitution. |
| Soy Foods | Products made from soybeans such as miso, tofu, tempeh, natto, tamari, and soy sauce. |
| Suribachi | A serrated, glazed clay bowl or mortar. It is used with a pestle, called a surikogi, for grinding and puréeing foods. |
| Sushi | A traditional Japanese dish consisting of rice seasoned with vinegar and served with various vegetables, sea vegetables, seafood, or pickles. In addition to spiral rounds, sushi can be prepared in several other styles. |
| Sushi Mat | A small bamboo mat used to roll up nori-maki sushi or to cover bowls and dishes to keep food warm. |
| Sweet Rice | Also called waxy or glutonous, this rice is slightly sweeter to the taste than regular rice and used in a variety of regular and holiday dishes. |
| Tahini | A thick, smooth paste made from ground sesame seeds. |

| | |
|---|---|
| Tamari | Traditional, naturally made soy sauce as distinguished from refined, chemically processed soy sauce. Also known as organic or natural shoyo. A stronger, wheat-free soy sauce called real or genuine tamari, a by-product of making miso, is used for special dishes. Tamari soy sauce is used for daily cooking. |
| Tekka | Condiment made from hatcho miso, sesame oil, burdock, lotus root, carrot, and ginger root. It cooks down to a black powder when sautéed on a low heat for several hours. |
| Tempeh | A traditional Indonesian soy food made from split soybeans, water, and special bacteria. Fermenting the soybeans for about one day can make tempeh, or it can be purchased ready-made in many natural food stores. High in protein and with a rich dynamic taste, tempeh is used in soups, stews, sandwiches, casseroles, and a variety of other dishes. |
| Tofu | Soybean curd made from soybeans and nigari. |
| Udon | Japanese whole-wheat noodles. |
| Umeboshi Plums | A salted, pickled plum aged for several years. |
| Umeboshi Vinegar | Liquid that umeboshi plums are aged in. Also known as ume-su. |
| Wakame | A long, thin green sea vegetable used in making miso soup. |
| Whole Foods | Food in its raw, unrefined, and unprocessed form, such as brown rice or whole wheat. Also known as natural foods. |
| Whole Grains | Unrefined cereal grains to which nothing has been added or subtracted in milling except the inedible outer hull. |
| Wild Rice | A wild cereal grass native to North America. |
| Yang | One of the two fundamental energies of the universe. Yang refers to the relative tendency of contraction, centripetally, density, heat, light, and other qualities. Yang energy tends to go down and inward in the vegetable kingdom. Yang predominates in small compact grains such as brown rice, millet, and buckwheat; in root vegetables; and in sea salt, miso, and tamari soy sauce. Its complementary and antagonistic energy is Yin. |
| Yin | One of the two fundamental energies of the universe. Yin refers to the relative tendency of expansion, growth, centrifugally, diffusion, cold, darkness, and other qualities. Yin energy tends to go up and outward in the vegetable kingdom. Yin energy predominates in large whole grains (such as corn, oats, and barley), leafy green vegetables, oils, nuts, fruits, and most liquids. Its complementary and antagonistic energy is Yang. |

# NOTES

**Stories and Portraits**

[1] Wepman, Marquita. "Menopause: A Transition Not an End." *Macrobiotic News* May/June 1996.

**Chapter One / The Menopausal Passage**

[2] Reuben, David. *Everything You Always Wanted to Know About Sex, But Were Afraid to Ask.* NY, NY: Bantam Books, 1969.

[3] McKinlay, Sonja and McKinlay, John. "The Massachusetts Women's Health Study; an epidemiologic investigation of menopause." *J Am Med Women's Assoc* Mar/Apr 1995. 50(2):45–49, 63.

[4] Northrup, Christiane. *Women's Bodies, Women's Wisdom.* NY, NY: Bantam Books, 1998. 443–444.

[5] Perry, S. and O'Hanlan, K. *Natural Menopause.* Reading, MA: Addison-Wesley Publishing, 1992. 9.

[6] Perry, S. and O'Hanlan, K. *Natural Menopause.* Reading, MA: Addison-Wesley Publishing, 1992. 17.

[7] Lee, John. "Is natural progesterone the missing link in osteoporosis prevention and treatment?" *Medical Hypothesis* 1991. 35:316–318.

Lee, John. "Osteoporosis Reversal: The Role of Progesterone." *International Clinical Nutrition Review* 1990. 10(3):384–391.

Lee, John. "Significance of molecular configuration specificity; the case of progesterone and osteoporosis." *Townsend Letter for Doctors* June 1993. 558–562.

[8] Northrup, Christiane. *Women's Bodies, Women's Wisdom.* NY, NY: Bantam Books, 1998. 430–484.

[9] Messina, Mark, et al. "Soy intake and cancer risk: a review of the in vitro and in vivo data." *Nutr Cancer*, 1994. 21:113–131.

[10] Karpman, Leonard, MD. "Phytoestrogens and Corporate America." *San Francisco Medicine* Sept 2002. 9.

[11] Kurzer, Mindy. "Diet, Estrogen and Cancer." *Contemporary Nutrition* 7(17):1–2.

[12] Weed, Susun. *New Menopausal Years the Wise Woman Way*. Woodstock, NY: Ash Tree Publishing, 2002. 102.

[13] Willett, W.C., et al. "Dietary flavonols and flavonol-rich foods intake and the risk of breast cancer." *International Journal of Cancer* April 2005. 114(4):628–633.

[14] Eastell, R. and Lambert, H. "Strategies for skeletal health in the elderly." *Proc Nutr Soc* May 2002. 62(2):173–189.

[15] Hurwitz, B., et al. "Putting the woman in her place." *British Medical Journal*, Feb 1989. 298(6669)299–305.

[16] Proulx, W. and Weaver, C. "Calcium absorption from plants." *The Soy Connection* Spring 1994. 2(2):1–4.

[17] Eastell, R. and Lambert, H. "Strategies for skeletal health in the elderly." *Proc Nutr Soc* May 2002. 62(2):173–180.

**Chapter Two / Benefits Of Macrobiotics For The Menopausal Passage**

[18] Molvig, Dianne. "41 ways to cope with menopause naturally." *Natural Health* May 1995. 25(3):88–94.

[19] Sparber, A., et al. "Use of complementary medicine by adult patients participating in cancer clinical trials." *Oncology Nurses Forum* 2000. 27(4):623–630.

# REFERENCES

Adlercreutz, Herman, et al. "Lignans and flavonoids inhibit aromatase enzyme in human preadipocytes." *J Steroid Biochem Mol Bio*, 1994. 50:205–212.

Austen, Haillie. *The Heart Of The Goddess*. CA: Wigbow Press, 1990.

Brawer, Rosen. *Making Their Mark*. NY, NY: Abbeville Press, 1989.

Broude, Garrard. *The Power Of Feminist Art*. NY: Abrams Press, 1994.

Chadwick, Whitney. *Women, Art And Society*. London England: Thames and Hudson, 1990.

Colbin, Annemarie. *Food And Our Bones*. NY, NY: Plume Books, 1998.

Follingstad, Alvin. "Estriol, the Forgotten Estrogen?" *The Journal of the American Medical Association*, 1978. 239(1), 29–30.

Freeman, Sarah. "Menopause without HRT: Complementary therapies." *Contemporary Nurse Practitioner*, Jan/Feb 1995. 40–49.

George, Demetra. *Mysteries of the Dark Moon*. San Francisco, CA: HarperCollins, 1992.

Gittleman, Ann Louise. *Super Nutrition for Menopause*. NY, NY: Pocket Books, 1993.

Goodman, Ellen. "Health Risks for Women Never More Confusing." *Minneapolis Star Tribune*, June 18, 1995. 17A.

Gouma-Peterson, Thalia, and Mathews, Patricia. "The Feminist Critique of Art History." *Art Bulletin*, 1989. 69(3): 326–357.

Hanley, Jesse. *Menopause: Dispelling the Myths, Telling the Truth, Exploring the Possibilities*. California: VHS-Producer Moondancer, 1993.

Hargrove, Joel, et al. "Menopausal hormone replacement therapy with continuous daily oral micronized estradiol and progesterone." *Obstetrics & Gynecology*, 1989. 73:606–612.

Hemminki, Nina and Shivo, Tinikka. "A review of postmenopausal hormone therapy recommendations: potential for selection bias." *Obstetrics & Gynecology*, 1993. 82(6) 1021–1028.

Hickock, Lee R., et al. "A comparison of esterified estrogens with and without methyl testosterone: effects on endometrial histology and serum lipoproteins in postmenopausal women." *Obstetrics & Gynecology*, 1993. 82(6): 919–924.

Klein, Richard. *The Green World.* NY, NY: HarperCollins, 1987.

Kurzer, Mindy and Campell, Deborah. "Flavonoid inihibition of aromatase enzyme activity in human predipocytes." *J Steroid Biochem Mol Bio*, 1993. 46(3):381–388.

Kurzer, Mindy, et al. "Effects of flax seed ingestion on the menstrual cycle." *J of Clin Endocrinology and Metabolism*, 1993. 77(5):1215–1219.

Kurzer, Mindy. "Estrogenic and anti-estrogenic effect of phyto-chemicals in soybeans and flaxseed." *Nutri-News*, 1995. 11–12.

Kurzer, Mindy, et al. "Urinary lignan and isoflavonoid excretion in premenopausal women consuming flaxseed powder." *American Journal of Clinical Nutrition*, 1994. 60:122–128.

Mason, Jerry. *The Family of Woman.* NY: Putnam Publishing, 1983.

Northrup, Christiane. *Menopause, A Time of Knowing.* Boulder, CO: Sounds True, 1993.

Nobel, Vicki. *Shakti Women.* New York, NY: HarperCollins, 1991.

Ojeda, Linda. *Menopause Without Medicine.* CA: Hunter House, 2000.

Raz, Raul and Stamm, Walter. "A controlled trial of intravaginal estriol in postmenopausal women with recurrent urinary tract infections." *The New England Journal Of Medicine*, 1993. 329(11):753–756.

Sheehy, Gail. *The Silent Passage: Menopause.* New York, NY: Pocket Books, 1993.

Taylor, Dena, et al. *Women of the 14th Moon.* Freedom, CA: Crossing Press, 1991.

Wilson, Robert. *Feminine Forever.* New York, NY: Evans and Company, 1966.

# RESOURCES

Now that you are aware of the importance of macrobiotics, the resources listed here will provide you with the information you need to maintain this healthy way of life. You will find natural and organic food resources, counselors, and study centers in this section. There is not enough room, however, for all of the wonderful people working in this field for a sustainable future. Please visit the following websites for additional information:

www.macrobioticdirectory.com
www.worldmacro.org
www.cybermacro.com

## Ann Louise Gittleman, PhD, CNS

The First Lady of Nutrition
12 Raymond Drive
Wilbraham, MA 01095
*Business and Operations Manager:*
Stuart K. Gittleman
*Phone:* 413-525-0044
*Fax:* 209-396-3919
*Email:* stuart@annlouise.com
*Website:* www.annlouise.com

In *Hot Times: How to Eat Well, Live Healthy, and Feel Sexy During the Change* (Avery, 2005), Ann Louise Gittleman demystifies menopause and discusses the most pressing menopausal issues for women today, including stress, osteoporosis, heart disease, breast cancer, diabetes, and hypothyroidism. Dr. Gittleman is also the best-selling author of **The Fat Flush Plan** and **Before the Change**.

## Amberwaves

PO Box 487
Becket, MA 01223
*President:* Alex Jack
*Phone:* 413-623-0012
*Fax:* 413-623-6042
*Email:* info@amberwaves.org
*Website:* www.amberwaves.org

*Amberwaves is a network of individuals, families, and businesses devoted to preserving rice, wheat, and other essential foods from the threat of genetic engineering, as well as keeping America and the planet beautiful. It publishes related books and a magazine. Alex Jack and his wife Gale—macrobiotic teachers, counselors, and writers—offer guidance on personal and family health in the Amberwaves newsletter, the "Macrobiotic Path."*

## Brooke Medicine Eagle

61529 Highway 93
Ste. A PMB 401
Polson, MT 59860
*Phone:* 406-883-4686
*Website:* www.MedicineEagle.com

*Brooke Medicine Eagle provides Native American teachings, ceremonies, soul retrieval, and shamanic illuminations. She offers private consultations and spiritual retreats, as well as teaching and singing tapes, books on the mysteries of moon time, and aboriginal and natural living skills.*

## Christiane Northrup, MD

PO Box 199
Yarmouth, ME 04096
*Fax:* 207-846-8953
*Email:* requests@drnorthrup.com
*Website:* www.drnorthrup.com

*Dr. Christiane Northrup, a visionary in the field of women's health and wellness, is the best-selling author of **The Wisdom of Menopause** (Bantam, 2006), **Women's Bodies, Women's Wisdom,** (Bantom, 2006), and **Mother-Daughter Wisdom** (Bantom, 2005). Dr. Northrup offers a monthly e-letter, "Women's Health Wisdom," and an exclusive print newsletter, "The Dr. Christiane Northrup Newsletter." Her work has been featured on the Oprah Winfrey Show, the Today Show, and NBC Nightly News with Tom Brokaw.*

## Christina Cooks

Christina Pirello
243 Dickinson Street
Philadelphia, PA 19147
*Phone:* 800-939-3909
*Fax:* 215-551-9498

*Email:* christinacooks@comcast.net
*Website:* www.christinacooks.com

*Christina Pirello takes the mystery out of preparing whole foods and presents a holistic approach to self-care with a liberal sprinkling of fun to her books **Cooking The Whole Foods Way, Cook Your Way To The Life You Want, Christina Cooks,** and **Glow.** She presents natural cooking through her TV show and has a bi-monthly magazine titled **Christina Cooks.***

## Denny Waxman

1223 South 2nd Street
Philadelphia, PA 19147
*Phone:* 215-271-1858
*Email:* info@dennywaxman.com
*Website:* www.DennyWaxman.com

*Denny Waxman is a senior macrobiotic counselor, educator, and author, and has active macrobiotic counseling practices in Philadelphia, PA and New York, NY. He is the founder, director, and a core faculty member for the Strengthening Health Institute, and author of **The Great Life Handbook** and **Recalled by Life**.*

## EarthSave International

PO Box 96
New York, NY 10108
*Phone:* 800-362-3648
*Fax:* 718-228-2491
*Email: information@earthsave.org*
*Website: www.earthsave.org*

*EarthSave supplies planet-friendly and life-sustaining information through a newsletter and website. Local EarthSave chapters provide educational materials and hold activities such as video showings and healthy food festivals.*

## Eden Foods, Inc.

701 Tecumseh Road
Clinton, MI 49236
*Phone:* 888-424-EDEN
*Fax:* 517-456-7025 (orders only)
*Website:* www.edenfoods.com

*Eden Foods provides quality, organic, macrobiotic foods that can be found at discerning food stores and co-ops, as well as on its website.*

## French Meadow Bakery & Café

2610 Lyndale Avenue South
Minneapolis, MN 55408
*Contact:* Lynn R. Gordon
*Phone:* 877-NO-YEAST
*Website:* www.frenchmeadow.com

*French Meadow Bakery offers the most nutritious and best-tasting certified organic sourdough breads, including Women's Bread and other award-winning items, nationwide. French Meadow Café is equally committed to serving locally grown organic foods, paying attention to the body's needs and the seasons, and supporting the environment and social justice unconditionally.*

## George Ohsawa Macrobiotic Foundation

Carl and Julia Ferre
PO Box 3998
Chico, CA 95927
*Phone:* 800-232-2372
*Fax:* 530-566-9768
*Email:* gomf@earthlink.net
*Website:* www.gomf.macrobiotic.net

*The George Ohsawa Macrobiotic Foundation publishes macrobiotic books,*
*the Macrobiotics Today magazine, and provides services to the macrobiotic community around the world.*

## Gold Mine Natural Food Company

Jean M. Richardson, President
7805 Arjons Drive
San Diego, CA 92126
*Phone:* 800-475-3363 (orders)
        858-537-9830 (customer service)
*Email:* sales@goldminenaturalfood.com
*Website:* www.goldminenaturalfood.com

*Gold Mine offers a full line of the highest quality macrobiotic foods to order.*

## Holistic Holiday at Sea

Sandy Pukel
434 Aragon Ave.
Coral Gables, Fl 33134
*Phone:* 305-725-0081
*Fax:* 305-447-3073
*Email:* oakfeed1@aol.com
*Website:* www.atasteofhealth.org

*Sandy Pukel has been a state licensed nutritional counselor for over twenty-five years. His yearly cruise, the Holistic Holiday at Sea: A Voyage to Well-Being, is a vacation with a purpose. It combines fun and relaxation with an incredible opportunity to learn from some of the world's most dynamic and experienced healers in holistic health.*

## John Kozinski's Elements of Health

*Phone:* 413-623-5925
*Fax:* 413-623-9909
*Email:* macrobiotic@macrobiotic.com
*Website:* www.macrobiotic.com

John Kozinski, MEA, has been a macrobiotic teacher, counselor, and researcher for thirty years. He is a senior faculty member at the Kushi Institute in Becket, Massachusetts, and maintains a private teaching and counseling practice traveling monthly to a number of US locations. He has aided thousands of people in the recovery of such diverse ailments as cancer, heart disease, pre-menstrual syndrome, endometriosis, urinary tract infections, and chronic fatigue syndrome.

## Kushi Institute

PO Box 7
Becket, MA 01223
Phone: 800-975-8744
Fax: 413-623-5741
Email: programs@kushiinstitute.org
Website: www.kushiinstitute.org

Founded by preeminent macrobiotic authority Michio Kushi, the Kushi Institute campus is located in the beautiful Berkshire Mountains of western Massachusetts. Experienced faculty guide participants in programs geared for a variety of interests including health recovery support; teacher, counselor, and cook certification; weekend workshops; conferences; and more.

## Kushi Store

Becket, MA 01223
Phone: 800-645-8744
Fax: 413-623-2315
Email: customerservice@kushistore.com
Website: www.kushistore.com

The Kushi Store mail-order division offers the highest quality macrobiotic foods plus cookware, gifts, and books, delivered to your door.

## Macrobiotic Education for Health

Milenka "Mina" Dobic
2402A Sacada Circle
Carlsbad, CA 92009
Phone: 760-436-4499
Fax: 760-436-4499
Email: minadobic@adelphia.net
Website: www.minadobic.org

Milenka "Mina" Dobic is an international macrobiotic educator and counselor who teaches nutrition, macrobiotic cooking classes, and philosophy at the School of Healing Arts in San Diego. She also lectures worldwide, and counsels people both in person and over the Internet.

## The Macrobiotic Guide UK

Phone: 44 (0) 1689 896175
Email: mail@macrobiotics.co.uk
Website: www.macrobiotics.co.uk

The Macrobiotic Guide is an extraordinary site that has a non-judgmental approach and openness in encouraging the exploration of macrobiotic lifestyles.

## Marquita Wepman

Phone: 828-299-7999 (Mar-Dec)
         954-260-7912 (Dec-Mar)
Email: warrenwep@bellsouth.net

Marquita Wepman is a Kushi Institute graduate, a certified cooking teacher, and a member of the Macrobiotic Educators Association (MEA). She offers cooking instruction, diet and lifestyle counseling, and instructions on setting up and stocking a macrobiotic kitchen. Marquita gives classes at the Kushi Institute.

## Muso Company

*Phone:* +81-6-6316-6012
*Fax:* +81-6-6316-6016
*Website:* www.muso-intl.co.jp/english

*For the past thirty years, the Muso Company has been dedicated to selecting the best quality organic foods and supplying these items to customers throughout the world. It offers a wide variety of high quality macrobiotic specialties as well as natural and traditional foods and kitchen supplies.*

## Natural Gourmet Institute for Health and Culinary Arts

Annemarie Colbin, PhD
48 West 21st Street, 2nd floor
New York, NY 10010
*Phone:* 212-645-5170, ext. 0
*Website:* www.naturalgourmetschool.com

*The Institute offers a Chef's Training Program, public classes, events and retreats, friday night dinners, and nutritional consultations.*

## Peninsula Macrobiotic Community

First Baptist Church
305 North California Avenue
Palo Alto, CA 94301
*Phone:* 650-599-3320 for reservations
*Email:* GerardTL@aol.com (Gerard T. Lum)
*Website:* Peninsulamacro.org

*The community offers dinner menus, a newsletter, and more. Mondays at 6:30 PM, there are gourmet vegetarian dinners made by Chef Gary Alinder and after-dinner lectures or other events. Check the website or call for a full schedule.*

## The Rice House

Sheldon and Ginat Rice
Mevo Betar, Israel 99878

*Phone:* 9722-534-0550
*Email:* Shelgin@netvision.net.il

*Sheldon and Ginat Rice began practicing macrobiotics in the early 1980s, and have experienced both their own healing and that of many clients. Ginat is a macrobiotic teacher, counselor, and shiatsu practitioner; Sheldon excels in numerology and has written a textbook called* **Getting to Know You.** *Together they offer a home-based macrobiotic live-in program of study and guidance in the macrobiotic way of life in Israel.*

## Self-Healing Australia

21 O'Hara St.
Marrickville NSW 2204 Australia
*Contact:* Issi Aaron
*Phone:* (+61 2) 9558 8111
*Email:* issi@self-healing.com.au
*Website:* www.self-healing.com.au

*Self-Healing Australia is a natural therapy website offering reference material for a range of modalities, as well as Zen shiatsu and holistic counseling services. It also includes the Macrobiotic Handbook for All Seasons, a free online resource containing an introduction to macrobiotics, twelve yoga poses for all seasons, and over seventy-five delicious and nutritious macrobiotic recipes with an interactive glossary of ingredients.*

## Strengthening Health Institute

Café, Store, and Educational Facility
Denny and Susan Waxman,
Founders and Directors
1149 North 3rd Street
Philadelphia, PA 19123
*Phone:* 215-271-0158
*Email:* info@strengthenhealth.org
*Website:* www.strengthenhealth.org

*The Strengthening Health Institute is a broad-*

based macrobiotic center integrating the work of like-minded teachers. The center offers day classes, dinner lectures, free lectures, five-day Strengthening Health Intensives, and a one-year program.

## Susan Krieger, Licensed Acupuncturist, MS

19 East 65th Street, Suite #1B
NY, New York 10021
*Phone:* 212-242-4217
*Email:* info@susankriegerhealth.com
*Website:* www.susankriegerhealth.com

*Susan Krieger, an internationally recognized practitioner of a variety of healing arts, offers lectures, workshops, and courses in topics including wholistic health and body-mind medicine.*

## US Food and Drug Administration

Center for Food Safety and Applied Nutrition
5600 Fishers Lane
Rockville, Maryland 20857
*Phone:* 800-SAFEFOOD
*Website:* www.cfsan.fda.gov/seafood1.html

*You can visit this website or call this tollfree number weekdays from 10 AM to 4 PM ET for advisory information regarding mercury and other contaminants for fish and seafood.*

## Utne Magazine

*Phone:* 800-736-UTNE (for subscription)
612-338-5040 (editorial and management offices)
*Website:* www.utne.com

*Utne, a leading voice in independent media, offers stories ranging from the environment to the economy and from politics to pop culture by utilizing thousands of indie publications, websites, blogs, books, films, and other off-the-beaten-path sources.*

## Wise Women Center

Susun Weed
PO Box 64
Woodstock, NY 12498
*Phone:* 845-246-8081
*Website:* www.herbshealing.com,
www.menopause-metamorphosis.com

*Susun Weed is the author of five best-selling women's health books, with topics including menopause, breast health, cancer prevention, childbearing and fertility, personal empowerment, and spirit healing. Her website offers free information on how to make nourishing herbal infusions, sources for herbs, and classes and workshops for the menopausal passage.*

## Women's International Pharmacy

2 Marsh Court
Madison, WI 53718
*Phone:* 800-279-5708
*Fax:* 608-221-7819
*Email:* info@womensinternational.com
*Website:* www.womensinternational.com

*Women's International Pharmacy is a compounding pharmacy dedicated to focusing on the patient's individual needs.*

## Yoga Macro

Karin Stephan
5 Frost Street
Cambridge, MA 02140
*Phone:* 617-497-0218
*Email:* KarinStephanYoga@aol.com
*Website:* www.yogamacro.com

*Karin Stephan offers lessons, workshops, and classes on yoga based on the teachings of B.K.S. Iyengar and the fundamentals of Oriental medicine. She also holds yoga/macrobiotic vacations at sea-side resorts around the world.*

# RECOMMENDED READINGS

Belleme, John and Belleme, Jan. *The Miso Book: The Art of Cooking with Miso*. Garden City Park, NY: Square One Publishers, 2006.

Carpenter, Ruth Ann and Finley, Carrie E. *Healthy Eating Every Day*. Champaign, IL: Human Kinetics, 2005.

Colbin, Annemarie. *The Natural Gourmet*. New York, NY: Balantine Books, 1989.

Gittleman, Ann Louise. *Hot Times: Eat Well, Live Healthy, Feel Sexy During the Change*. New York, NY: Avery, 2005.

Esko, Wendy and Kushi, Aveline. *Introducing Macrobiotic Cooking: A Primer and Cookbook*. Garden City Park, NY: Square One Publishers, 2006.

Jack, Gale. *Women's Health Guide*. Becket, MA: One Peaceful World Press, 1997.

Kushi, Aveline. *The Complete Guide To Macrobiotic Cooking*. New York, NY: Warner Books, 1985.

Kushi, Aveline with Esko, Wendy. *The Changing Seasons Cookbook*. New York, NY: Avery Publishing Group, 1985/2003.

Kushi, Michio. *The Dō-In Way: Gentle Exercises to Liberate the Body, Mind, and Spirit*. Garden City Park, NY: Square One Publishers, 2006.

Kushi, Michio. *Your Body Never Lies: The Complete Book of Oriental Diagnosis*. Garden City Park, NY: Square One Publishers, 2006.

Kushi, Michio and Jack, Alex. *The Macrobiotic Path to Total Health*. New York, NY: Balantine Books, 2003.

Kushi, Michio with Marc Van Cauwenberghe. *Macrobiotic Home Remedies*. Garden City Park, NY: Square One Publishers, 2007.

McCarty, Meredith. *Fresh from a Vegetarian Kitchen*. New York, NY: St. Martin's Press, 1989.

Melina, Vesanto, et al. *Food Allergy Survival Guide*. Summertown, TN: Healthy Living Publications, 2004.

Melina, Vesanto and Davis, Brenda. *The New Becoming Vegetarian*. Summertown, TN: Healthy Living Publications, 2003.

Ohsawa, Lima. *The Art of Just Cooking*. Brookline, MA: Autumn Press, 1975.

Pirello, Christina. *Cooking the Whole Foods Way*. New York, NY: Berkley Publishing Group, 1997.

Porter, Jessica. *The Hip Chick's Guide to Macrobiotics*. New York, NY: Avery Publishing Group, 2004.

Robbins, John. *The Food Revolution: How Your Diet Can Help Save Your Life and Our World*. Berkeley, CA: Conari Press, 2001.

Schlosser, Eric. *Fast Food Nation: The Dark Side of the All-American Meal*. Boston, MA: Houghton Mifflin, January 2001.

Turner, Kristina. *The Self-Healing Cookbook*. Crass Valley, CA: Earthtones Press, 1987/2002.

Walden, Patricia and Sparrowe, Linda. *The Women's Book of Yoga and Health*. Boston, MA: Shambhala Publications, 2002.

# ABOUT THE AUTHOR

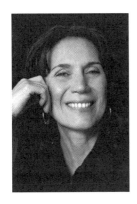

*Gabriele Kushi* is a certified macrobiotic health educator, counselor, and cooking teacher. For more than thirty years, she has helped people from all over the world and all walks of life become healthier and more self-reliant by choosing natural foods and sustainable lifestyles. She has published numerous articles on healing with natural foods, and has spoken about macrobiotics on radio talk shows. She is a member of the Macrobiotic Educators Association and serves on the advisory board of Earth Save International. Gabriele also holds a BFA in photography, and her fine art has been exhibited in Minnesota. She teaches in Germany and the United States.

Be sure to visit *www.kushiskitchen.com* for more information on:

| | |
|---|---|
| Counseling and coaching services | Educational services and schools |
| Cooking classes | Seminars |
| Recipes | Books and tapes |
| Chef services | Resources for ordering natural foods and herbs |
| Workshops | |

# INDEX

## I

Ingredients for recipes, 105–106
Insomnia. *See* Symptoms, menopausal.
*International Journal of Cancer*, 29
Irritability. *See* Symptoms, menopausal.

## J

*Journal of the American Medical Association*, 25

## K

Kudzu, 49
Kudzu Sauce, Pan-Fried Tofu in, 78
Kushi, Aveline, 1, 8–9, 45, 46
Kushi, Michio, 46
Kushi Institute, 46

## L

Land vegetables, 50
Leafy Green Vegetable Roll, 83
Legumes, 50
Libido, loss of. *See* Symptoms, menopausal.
Licata, Michelle, 98
Lignan, 27
Liquids, 50
Luteinizing Hormone (LH), 24

## M

Macrobiotics
    activities and exercises for, 45
    general meals for, 48
    introduction to, 45–48
    philosophy of, 47
    recipes for, 66–104
    teachings of, 47
Magnesium, 31
Maki Roll, Sushi, 100
Mashed potatoes, substituting for, 68

McKinley, John, 19
McKinley, Sonja, 19
Mead, Margaret, 23
Meals, preparing, 48. *See also* Ingredients
    for recipes; Recipes.
Meat, eating, 22, 49, 120
Medicine Eagle, Brooke, 12–13
Menarche, definition of, 21
Menopause
    definition of, 21
    as enlightenment, 61, 119
    and herbal relief of symptoms, 28, 111
    and naturally easing symptoms, 21
    stages of, 23
    *See also* Symptoms, menopausal.
Menstruation
    end of, 21, 24
    irregular, 21, 23
    *See also* Personal stories.
Midlife issues, 29–32
Millet a la Mashed Potato, 68
Miso
    health benefits of, 71
    relationship of, to estrogen/breast cancer,
        29
    relationship of, to lessened menopausal
        symptoms, 26, 28
Miso Soup, 71
Monroe, Marilyn, 63–64
Mood swings. *See* Symptoms, menopausal.
Morrow, Monica, 25

## N

National Museum of American History, the,
    46
Natural food
    calcium content of, 32
    recipes, 65–104

## YOUR BODY NEVER LIES

The Complete Book of Oriental Diagnosis

Michio Kushi

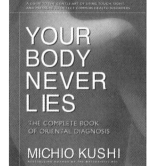

Too often, conventional medicine fails to detect illness. But Oriental diagnosis, an ancient holistic system of knowledge, can often discover physical problems even before they arise. Beginning with an explanation of the principles of Oriental medicine—touching, "seeing," and pressure— *Your Body Never Lies* helps you understand this natural, noninvasive approach to detecting sickness.

*Your Body Never Lies* provides an in-depth exploration of the components of seeing. This includes a description of deviations in facial features, skin, and extremities; irregularities in posture, movement, and mental states; and more. Within this unique intuitive system is the power to detect the body's warning signs and avert serious illness, including cancer and heart disease.

Western medical practice often focuses on a specific body part, symptom, or ailment, ignoring the totality and interconnectedness of the human body. *Your Body Never Lies* is a complete guide to Oriental diagnosis, a revolutionary—yet centuries-old—way to detect and prevent disease, and to preserve health and biological harmony.

---

*January 2007 • $17.95 US / $26.95 CAN • 288 pages • 7.5 x 9-inch quality paperback • ISBN 0-7570-0267-6*

---

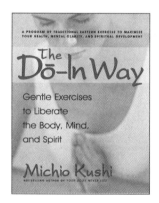

## THE DŌ-IN WAY

Gentle Exercises to Liberate the Body, Mind, and Spirit

Michio Kushi

Dō-In is an ancient traditional exercise for the cultivation of physical health, mental serenity, and spirituality. Over the last 5,000 years, it has served as the origin of such well-known disciplines as shiatsu, acupuncture, yogic exercises, moxibustion, and meditation. Literally meaning to pull and stretch, Dō-In originated as a way of achieving longevity and attaining the highest potential of mental and spiritual development. This exercise offers release from physical sickness, confusion, and intellectual and social disharmony.

Dō-In techniques are a series of successive motions designed to harmonize body systems. *The Dō-In Way* details the fundamental aspects of this exercise, which involves breathing, self-massage, and posture, and manipulation to stimulate bodily systems. The gentle application of pressure on the body's meridians corresponds directly with physical processes, and allows for the conditioning and stimulation of internal organs.

Dō-In is a simple, gentle exercise for achieving oneness between the self and the external world. *The Dō-In Way* is a comprehensive handbook to this basic, primal form of exercise—an ancient system of movement designed to enhance physical, mental, and spiritual health.

---

*$15.95 US / $23.95 CAN • 224 pages • 7.5 x 9-inch quality paperback • Exercise/Health/Macrobiotics • ISBN 0-7570-0268-4*

# MACROBIOTIC HOME REMEDIES

## Your Guide to Traditional Healing Techniques

Michio Kushi with Marc Van Cauwenberghe, MD

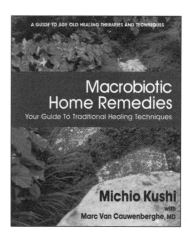

It is simple in its approach, and powerful in its effect—a diet of natural foods and the use of noninvasive home remedies, designed to eliminate disease symptoms and strengthen the body's own healing powers. In the past, these remedies were passed from generation to generation by word of mouth. Today, they are embodied by the macrobiotic movement.

*Macrobiotic Home Remedies* is a comprehensive self-help guide to hundreds of effective natural healing methods that can be used alone or in conjunction with more standard remedies—methods that heal without drugs or invasive treatments. The book is divided into four sections. It begins by explaining the healing concepts of macrobiotics. Part Two then provides an A-to-Z reference to over two hundred common health disorders, with helpful suggestions for relief. Part Three details the numerous techniques and therapies suggested in Part Two. Part Four presents over two hundred healing recipes referred to throughout the book.

For years, Michio Kushi has dedicated his life to teaching the macrobiotic way to better health. Now his knowledge is available to you and your family in this complete guide to the art of healing.

*January 2007 • $17.95 US / $22.50 CAN • 288 pages • 7.5 x 9-inch quality paperback • ISBN 0-7570-0269-2*

---

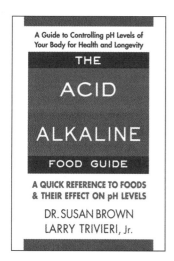

# THE ACID-ALKALINE FOOD GUIDE

## A Quick Reference to Foods & Their Effect on pH Levels

Susan E. Brown, PhD, CCN and Larry Trivieri, Jr.

The last five years have seen an explosion of best-selling acid/alkaline-based diet books—books on weight loss, on diabetes management, and more. While thousands of people are trying to balance their body's pH level, until now, they have had to rely on the very limited food guides contained in these books. Now, health experts Dr. Susan E. Brown and Larry Trivieri have created a complete resource for people who want to widen their food choices. *The Acid-Alkaline Food Guide* offers dieters an easy-to-follow guide to the most common foods that influence the body's pH levels.

The book begins by explaining how the acid/alkaline environment of the body is influenced by foods. It then presents a list of thousands of foods and their acid/alkaline effects—effects that, in many cases, are surprising. Included are informative insets that can assist you in choosing the best foods for your needs.

The first book of its kind, *The Acid-Alkaline Food Guide* will quickly become the resource you turn to at home, in restaurants, and whenever you want to select a food that can help you reach your health and dietary goals.

*$7.95 US / $9.95 CAN • 160 pages • 4 x 7-inch quality paperback • Health/Nutrition • ISBN 0-7570-0280-3*

# THE MISO BOOK
## The Art of Cooking with Miso
### John and Jan Belleme

For centuries, the preparation of miso has been considered an art form in Japan. Through a time-honored double-fermentation process, soybeans and grains are transformed into this wondrous food, which is a flavorful addition to a variety of dishes and a powerful medicinal. Scientific research has supported miso's use as an effective therapeutic aid in the prevention and treatment of heart disease, certain cancers, radiation sickness, and hypertension.

Part One of this comprehensive guide begins with miso basics—its types and uses. A chapter called "Miso Medicine" then details this superfood's healing properties and role in maintaining good health. Easy directions for making miso at home are also found in Part One. Fascinating insets, including the authors' adventures in Japan, where they learned the art of miso-making from a miso master, round out this section. Part Two presents over 140 delectable, healthy recipes in which miso is used in dips, spreads, soups, stews, and so much more.

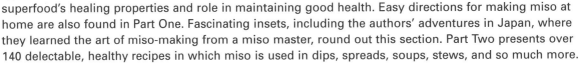

*$15.95 US / $23.95 CAN • 192 pages • 7.5 x 9-inch quality paperback • Cooking/Vegetarian/ Miso • ISBN 0-7570-0028-2*

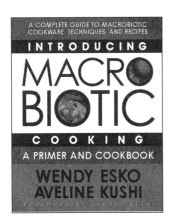

# INTRODUCING MACROBIOTIC COOKING
## A Primer and Cookbook
### Wendy Esko and Aveline Kushi

Since it first appeared, *Introducing Macrobiotic Cooking* has become a classic in the field as both a practical guide and an essential cookbook. Written by two world-renowned macrobiotic cooking instructors, this book has been used by thousands of people who are looking for a healthier approach to preparing meals. Whether you are a new or long-time follower of the macrobiotic lifestyle, *Introducing Macrobiotic Cooking* is the first place to turn for information on macrobiotics, for recipes, and for cooking techniques.

Fully illustrated, this book includes guidelines for setting up a macrobiotic kitchen, shopping for the highest-quality natural ingredients, and planning balanced meals. Over 200 easy-to-follow recipes are conveniently arranged according to food type, including complete sections on preparing whole grain, bean, vegetable, and sea vegetable dishes; baking whole grain breads; and preparing soyfoods like tofu and tempeh. Rounding out the recipes are special guidelines for preparing pickles, salads, seafood, and sugar-free natural desserts.

*January 2007 • $17.95 US / $26.95 CAN • 240 pages • 7.5 x 9-inch quality paperback • ISBN 0-7570-0270-6*